Think Right
Eat Right
Move Right

Think Right
Eat Right
Move Right

MARY PERIGOE

Book Guild Publishing
Sussex, England

This edition published in Great Britain in 2014 by
The Book Guild Ltd
The Werks
45 Church Road
Hove
East Sussex
BN3 2BE

First published in 2013 by The Incwadi Press, Cape Town, South Africa

Printed in Great Britain by
CPI Group (UK) Ltd, Croydon, CR0 4YY

A catalogue record for this book is available from
The British Library.

ISBN 978 1 909984 30 1

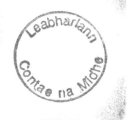

Think Right

means adopting balanced thoughts, attitudes, motives and beliefs which influence how and what we eat and how active we are mentally and physically

Eat Right

means balanced nutrition from fresh, natural foods and water, balancing intake with energy output to maintain a stable weight

Move Right

means balanced movement, practising correct posture, effective exercise and even breathing

FOREWORD

M ary's book is a *must have*. It's so comprehensive, easy to absorb and
a joy to read.

I love it as it covers all aspects of our health. It is full of helpful advice
which proves that if we take responsibility for ourselves, and give our
body and mind the TLC they need, we can stay in shape and independent
in later years.

It is no secret that I am not keen on "work outs", but I love Mary Perigoe's
exercise regime and I LOVE the results! My shape has improved – my
stomach muscles are now stronger and my back problems are less of an
issue (despite the fact I'm still endlessly moving furniture, lifting my
grandchildren and helping my husband, who weighs 16½ stone).

Mary's philosophy, which underpins the whole book, was developed as a
result of a personal crisis in her early life. This philosophy, which explores
such fundamental questions as the true meaning of life and health, has
been extremely helpful to me.

I want to have *Think Right, Eat Right, Move Right* by my side at all times,
and I wish I'd had this book years ago.

Mary Perigoe is an inspiration and an amazing example of all she advocates.

Susan Hampshire
London, January 2014

ACKNOWLEDGEMENTS

I am indebted to Mark, Arlene and Julia Stephenson for their invaluable assistance with the publication of the first edition of this book in Cape Town in 2013. I would also like to thank family and friends for their continuing support, Paul Newman for his useful suggestions and Sheila Tizzard for her exercise illustrations. A special thank you to Etan Ilfeld of Watkins Books for his belief in my book, also to Louisa Scott for the cover photos.

I am particularly grateful to Susan Hampshire for her enthusiastic encouragement and to everyone at The Book Guild for making our collaboration such an enjoyable experience.

Names have been changed where appropriate to preserve anonymity.

CONTENTS

Introduction

This is the story of my search for meaning in life, which led to a lifetime spent in the field of health and healing. In my twenties and thirties I faced difficulties with health, work and relationships that brought my life to crisis point and left me with an overwhelming need to understand how and why it had happened.

Unable to get satisfying answers from friends, doctors or the church, especially to my fundamental question – How can a good God allow such sickness, suffering and apparent inequalities to exist in the world? – my desperation drove me to explore unconventional therapies and philosophies little known at the time. I could never have foreseen what an exhilarating, mind expanding adventure I was embarking upon or the extent to which the exciting discoveries I would make would transform every area of my life: career (from medical social worker to natural health therapist), vastly increased vitality (mental, physical and emotional), happier relationships and, most of all, a philosophy free from dogma that answered all my questions.

I have written the book for people of any age who are on a similar quest, my aim being to provide straightforward guidelines to anyone seriously committed in their search to find health and fulfilment but struggling to make sense of their lives amidst the confusing and often conflicting influences in the world today.

Although this is essentially a self-help book rather than an autobiography, I have highlighted specific aspects of my personal life which had a direct bearing on the health and relationship problems I grappled with in my earlier years. By doing so I hope to encourage readers to engage in the step-by-step process I followed in order to overcome similar problems they may be experiencing in their own lives.

I believe the three essentials for healthy, happy living are: Think Right, Eat Right, Move Right. That is, adopt balanced thoughts (attitudes, motives, beliefs), balanced nutrition (fresh natural foods and water, balancing intake with energy output), and balanced movement (posture, exercise, breathing). Most important of all is the need for positive thoughts, which undoubtedly influence how and what we eat and how active we are mentally and physically.

Throughout the book I have shared problems I faced and lessons learned to illustrate how readers can make practical use of my experiences in their own lives. I have included critical incidents that shaped my thinking and influenced my life choices to show how these events helped me build my philosophy and eventually led to the development of my home visiting, teaching and therapy practice.

The whole process of good health
Since medicine is concerned mainly with early detection and removing the signs of disease, we have little idea of what constitutes perfect health. But it is a mistake to accept two to three colds a year, signs of arthritis over fifty and a life expectancy of seventy or so as normal, simply because these may represent the average. There are healthy, happy people well over 100 years, so why shouldn't we become one of them?

I believe health and vitality are two aspects of one whole. Whereas I would describe vitality as rhythmically flowing physical, mental, emotional and spiritual energies, I regard health as the harmonious relationship between body, mind and spirit.

Disease is not necessarily inevitable, but neither does it happen overnight. It is usually a gradual process and one which is reversible up to a certain degree of advancement.

Natural health, as a science, was practised by ancient civilisations and passed down over the centuries from the tenets formulated by Hippocrates, the Greek physician known as the Father of Medicine (c460–c375 BC).

Natural healing methods (practised by present-day naturopaths) are based on these three principles:

1. Most diseases are due to:
   - a lack of vital nutrients, either because insufficient foods are eaten or because somehow the body doesn't assimilate or use the nutrients properly.
   - too many waste products because of long-term smoking, drinking or excessive eating, too little exercise or rest, and too much emotional turmoil.

   The lack of food is happily rare in our Western society, but the lack of the right nutrients is all too common.

2. The vital energy force, the inner vitality, within each of us, can be used positively, and it can be supplemented by good food, good water, oxygen-rich air, and by the mental and spiritual inspiration that positive thinking can bring.

3. The body's own restorative forces can be revitalised and redirected when they have gone awry.

Acute diseases such as fevers, colds, diarrhoea, skin eruptions, inflammations and so on are attempts to get rid of waste material, and should not be suppressed. A temperature is actually nature's bonfire burning up the rubbish. Hippocrates is reputed to have said 'Give me a fever and I will cure every disease'. Of course, in severe cases this has to be controlled if there is fear of the life being in danger. Germs and bacteria are always present but only become active when the body, due to lowered vitality, becomes unable to dispose of waste in the normal way (through the skin, bowels, kidneys, lungs) and the waste clogs the system.

Dr René Dubos, a distinguished bacteriologist of the Rockefeller Institute for Medical Research, said that bacteria and viruses become dangerous only when the body's natural balance is disturbed.

Chronic diseases such as chronic bronchitis, circulatory problems, osteoarthritis, skin allergies, hay fever and sinusitis result from failure to implement the three essentials above; and/or continued suppression of acute diseases by the use of drugs and medicines that treat the symptoms only, pushing waste products further into the system. Drugs and medicines only stop the activities of bacteria and viruses temporarily, but kill antibodies, part of the body's natural defence mechanism. The danger is that we cannot forecast the long-term consequences of this type of treatment for future generations. The form which chronic disease takes depends on the constitution, and to some extent hereditary tendencies.

The resultant chronic condition does not describe a state of health (there have, for instance, been tennis champions and rowers such as Sir Steve Redgrave with diabetes and successful sportsmen who have had heart disease). The level of fitness we attain depends very much on individual aspirations and in some cases this could lead to unwise action. Someone with a gastric ulcer, for example, might be tempted to skip meals and work for long periods in order to gain mental satisfaction, but at the expense of aggravating the ulcer condition. Fitness relates to the ability to meet the demands of our environment – physical, emotional and mental – including our everyday activities and also emergencies such as accidents. So naturally, if we are fit we can lead a more productive life, work for longer periods without fatigue, and respond more efficiently when emergency situations do arise. From a physical standpoint this requires joint and muscle flexibility, strong even and sufficiently developed muscles capable of prolonged activity, efficient lungs and circulation, balance and co-ordination.

The causes of unfitness are similar to those of ill-health, although the emphasis may differ: negative attitudes, overweight, poor posture, lack of correct exercise, incorrect diet, smoking, and too much alcohol.

Home influences 1927–1932

Reflections on early childhood

In contemplating my early years I realised that the circumstances into which we are born, combined with our innate character traits, can both contribute to the cause of any problems we face and equally influence the solution. But as we grow up our initial situation tends to play a diminishing role as we take more responsibility for our self-development. That is why I have decided to share my early experiences in some detail to illustrate that, although the youth of today may face a different set of circumstances, the tools for self-help I have used throughout the years remain as effective as ever.

Readers may find it helpful to reflect on their own early years by acknowledging the positive aspects, gaining insight and working to resolve difficult issues which, inevitably, will lead to positive repercussions in their daily lives.

I was born into a modest, but stable home in an East Sussex village in 1927 and remained an only child until my sister arrived twelve years later.

At the age of three, I broke my arm and narrowly avoided serious damage to one eye. It happened in the local park where the village men played cricket. My mother helped prepare the teas and while she was busy, warned me not to go near the ponies that were free to roam there. But being true to my name (Mary, Mary quite contrary), I couldn't resist stroking one and not surprisingly he kicked me.

My father and I had happy times together. He loved to help me with jigsaw puzzles and I remember playing with him at the seaside (Winchelsea Beach) where my mother's family had a bungalow used at holiday times by the relatives during the summer.

Later on, when my sister arrived, May 1939, my mother found her easier to deal with. My sister was always laughing, which relaxed my mother's nervous system, whereas my mother and I were both highly-strung so we often clashed.

The incident with the pony was the first of many occasions that should have taught me there would be consequences from going against my mother's wishes as clearly she had my best interests at heart, but it would be some years before I learned to cope with emotional situations more logically and enjoy an easier relationship with my mother.

Parental background

My father and mother's families lived opposite each other in the village and my parents probably met on my maternal grandfather's tennis court. My paternal grandfather came to Northiam from Hastings to run the family building contractors' business. My mother was the second eldest of a large family (ten girls, one boy). Her older sister did not have any domestic skills and went to work in a bank, and my mother's job was to look after her younger siblings. Consequently she became a good homemaker and the best cook in the family. It was a pity that my mother had only a limited education at the local village school as she was intelligent and naturally talented, whereas my father was able to go to a good school. I always felt my mother suffered from an inferiority complex and maybe resented the fact that the younger members of her family had a better education. Mother was very musical and had her voice trained professionally, but had to teach herself to play the piano, violin and organ. For as long as I can remember she was the principal organist for the Northiam Chapel. She also had a good business head which was a great help to my father in his business. In addition, she wrote several booklets on local history, ran the Women's Institute choir for 21 years (winning many cups), compiled a scrapbook of the local W.I. with her older sister and achieved her ultimate ambition to found the Perigoe Workshop Museum which won an award during the European Architectural Heritage Year 1975. She was also interested in tracing the Perigoe family tree and discovered relatives all over the world, but mainly in Canada and Australia.

My father had three older sisters (one of whom died in childhood). Father served in the army in the First World War, but suffered from rheumatic fever so never went to the Front. It always appeared that his parents favoured his sisters and that he would have preferred to have followed a different career, but felt duty-bound to carry on the family business. He became a Methodist local preacher and held several other positions in the community that involved public speaking, all of which helped him overcome a nervous stutter. My father was sociable and well respected, but without my mother's practical support he might have gone bankrupt. He did not like office work so she practically had to tie him to his chair to do the estimating and send out the bills. Together they built up a reasonably prosperous business sufficient to send me and later my sister to public schools. But they worked incredibly hard with very little leisure time and were not able to enjoy a well-deserved retirement due to my father's premature death in 1963.

Pre-school years

From early childhood I struggled to control my emotional reactions and the problem continued into my twenties and thirties when I was forced to take stock and find a better way to deal with them. The problem surfaced initially when my mother and I clashed at meal times. Before I was of school age, I remember one of my aunts' tactless habit of remarking how pale and wan I looked, implying I wasn't being fed properly. This had the disastrous effect of my mother trying to fill me up with rich food, which I found difficult to digest (my father had gall bladder trouble later in life and I tended to take after him in health matters). Consequently, mealtimes became a battleground. I often refused to eat or, annoyingly, would put the food in my mouth but wouldn't swallow it. My mother was driven to distraction and tried to force the issue by hitting me with kindling sticks. To make matters worse I would then creep into the pantry between meals to pick at the food, inevitably getting caught in the process. Instinctively my body must have 'known' that food would not be digested properly in this emotional situation. Later on I learned that hormones and other chemicals secreted when in an emotional state interfere with the digestive juices. No wonder I tried to satisfy my hunger in the relative peace of the pantry.

School years: 1932–1945

First steps towards emotional independence

In 1932, when I was five, I started school and things improved dramatically. In my mind I can still see my two older cousins waiting at the top of the lane opposite our house to take me to school on my first day. I loved school from the outset. Getting away from my mother's overbearing fussiness, being able to channel my nervous energy through the lessons, and making new friends had a calming effect on me and my appetite returned with a vengeance, to my parents' great relief. As digestive juices can only flow normally in relaxed, pleasant conditions, it is important not to eat when angry, stressed, in a hurry or walking (as is common nowadays) since the food will not be chewed, digested and assimilated properly.

If this manner of eating becomes habitual it can lead to digestive problems, even unnecessary weight gain (from absorption into the body of incompletely digested food stuffs which cannot be utilised as nutrients) or in extreme cases as a gastric or duodenal ulcer. Comfort eating, using food (more often that which is high in sugar and fat) to satisfy emotional needs instead of dealing with the problem directly, is also common. I myself succumbed to this habit in the 1950s when feeling emotionally insecure and lacking in self-esteem. Later in life, as a therapist, I used this experience to help clients understand the link between emotion and food and the importance of finding balance in all areas of life.

Much later on, when facing challenging situations, I eventually found the inner strength to overcome fear of opposition and stand my ground. By working on areas where I lacked confidence, I gradually learned to face my fears and act positively one step at a time. Helped by the subsequent easing of tension and increase in energy, I was able to look objectively and accept myself, warts and all, as a friend. This gave me the confidence to express myself in difficult situations without losing emotional control, which had been impossible when I was younger. To know yourself better than anyone else does means there is nothing to fear from other people's criticism as their knowledge cannot match your own.

As a by-product, I found it easier to see through other people's emotional bias and understand their real needs, which was useful in my work as a therapist. As the saying goes, 'those who cannot stand alone, have nothing to give'. It's worth noting that to stand alone is not the same as being lonely. You cannot feel lonely for long if you are at one with yourself.

Boarding school: 1938–1945

Back in the 1930s, I continued my progression through primary school until I was ten years old. My cousins and other friends passed the 11+ exam and went to Rye Grammar School. I would have been happy to go there and mix more freely with the local community, but my parents had other ideas. They believed in the work ethic and strived to give me what they considered to be a good education by sending me to a Methodist boarding school, Farringtons in Chislehurst, Kent, over 50 miles away from home in January 1938 when I was ten and three-quarters, where I learned to mix with socially diverse groups including different nationalities and to become more able to stand on my own two feet. Initially I was very homesick, but I appreciated that my parents were doing their best for me. Leaving a sheltered home life in a small community was the first of many changes (sometimes sudden) that were to occur throughout my life, thrusting me into an increasingly wider world. It was helpful to learn many years later from an esoteric astrologer that having the planet Uranus very close to the Sun in the eighth house of my birth chart is indicative of shocks and sudden changes throughout life, which can be used as positive opportunities for transformation and renewal. Fortunately I discovered an innate ability to adapt to changing circumstances that has held me in good stead over the years.

In the village, a combination of my own shyness and my mother's protectiveness made it difficult for me to mix freely with the villagers, giving me the feeling of being different from others. This feeling continued at boarding school where I was catapulted overnight into an unfamiliar environment having to cope with a more extensive curriculum and mix with girls from wealthier backgrounds. I was also saddled with a broad Sussex accent not thought acceptable at that time, so the school decided to give me elocution lessons all of which made me feel socially inferior and added to my feeling of being different. Scholastically, I was ahead of the other girls but had not learned foreign languages at the village school so had to catch up with French and Latin. This wasn't too difficult as my classmates had only just started them. Maybe it was because the school wanted to encourage me that I was given the role of John Wesley (founder of Methodism) as a young boy in a school play. The girl who played my mother went on to become a Methodist Minister's wife and I met her again when her husband, Derrick Greaves, became the Minister of the Westminster Central Hall in the 1960s.

Prior to my change of school, my father's parents had died and we moved into the family home, a 14th century weatherboard house where my sister and brother-in-law live today. During this period, I remember listening to King Edward VIII's abdication speech on the radio. My mother became moodier than usual at this time, often not speaking for several days (though we could never understand the reason) leaving me fearful of emotional upsets which lasted into adulthood. I discovered bottles of Sanatogen (a nerve tonic) in a kitchen cupboard and later remember the doctor calling. Ever curious, I tried to listen at the keyhole, guessing rightly that my mother was pregnant although I was not told officially until it was obvious. My parents thought I would be jealous, but I was over the moon with excitement. We were convinced the baby was a boy and named him William John Pelham Perigoe (family names). But she was a girl! I was overjoyed to receive the news at school in my father's weekly letter. She was born on a Saturday, like me. Saturday's child works hard for his living – true of both of us.

Later that year war was declared. It was during the summer holidays (3 September, 1939) and the news was relayed by radio during the Sunday morning service in the Northiam Methodist Chapel. Almost immediately the air raid warning sounded, but of course, it was a false alarm. The local boys were soon enlisted into one of the armed forces. My father, at 46, was too old and would not have passed the medical on account of his history of rheumatic fever. Instead, he joined the Home Guard – local men who, unrealistically, were expected to stop Hitler's invasion when it came. At home we had to keep a packed bag under the bed so that we could evacuate quickly. It was thought that we were in the zone where the invasion forces would land, so only people with special passes could enter our area. Eventually the fear of invasion receded when Hitler invaded Russia instead. Every citizen was issued with a gas mask. It was widely feared that Hitler would use poisonous gas but fortunately he never did.

War time experiences 1939–1945

My war time experiences taught me to accept how transient and dangerous life can be. The Battle of Britain was fought overhead and we often saw shrapnel, planes, and parachutes falling from the sky. We had a dug-out in the garden where we could hide if things got too noisy. In the house we had another shelter under the dining room table where my sister and I slept during the roughest bombing periods. But I couldn't resist tickling her at night which usually woke her up and she retaliated by waking me at the crack of dawn.

My school was also in the firing line and was evacuated to Babbacombe, South Devon, almost 300 miles from home, but at the end of 1940 we were shocked by the news that the school was to close until after the war. The old headmistress had retired and the Governors did not wholly approve of the new one. In any case, the hotel we lived in was to be commandeered by the R.A.F. My friends' parents and mine quickly consulted and some of us found places for the new term at Queenswood, Hatfield, Hertfordshire, where I remained until the end of the war (1945).

I had been taught to play the piano from an early age by an aunt, my mother's youngest sister (a professional pianist) and I eventually passed all the piano exams. Ernest Read, a well known conductor and famous for his Saturday morning concerts for children, evacuated with his family to one of the school houses at Queenswood and I have many happy memories of his wildly enthusiastic sessions with the school choir and orchestra. He also taught me to play the organ. The only downside was that he was a chain smoker and had a nasty habit of dropping ash over his pupils. I was lucky enough to be in the Sanatorium (having mumps) with one of his daughters who brought in arm-loads of classical records, some of which are my favourites to this day.

In the holidays, on Sunday evenings when my father was out preaching, my mother would often give me an impromptu concert, singing or playing the piano or violin. At school I enjoyed playing piano duets with friends. One girl who was especially talented could play Grieg's Piano Concerto and later became Tony Armstrong-Jones's (Lord Snowdon) stepmother.

We listened to the radio in the school hall as the D-day landings took place (6 June 1944) and I was still at school on VE day, May 8th 1945. Before the war finally ended, Hitler played his last desperate card – the launch of his unmanned aircraft rockets known as V1s (nicknamed doodle-bugs) and V2s. The V2s were more feared because there was little or no warning of their approach. Our headmistress' house was demolished by a direct hit. Fortunately she was not there, but it didn't stop us girls giggling through a hymn that included the line 'The hosts of God encamp around the dwellings of the just ...'. We were thinking where were the hosts ... or wasn't she just!

During the worst of the blitz our beds were moved into the corridor, but V1 rockets couldn't reach beyond London and most of them dropped in the south-east of England. My father had a close shave when cycling through the village one day. He heard the familiar loud clattering sound as the rocket approached, followed by an eerie silence which signalled it was about to drop and explode. He quickly made for the nearest ditch in time to see the bomb explode in a field. In those days living with uncertainty was part of everyday life.

During 1944, two incidents influenced my future. One was the opportunity to watch operations performed by a school friend's father along with several other girls, some of whom had fainted or had to leave the operating theatre to be sick. I, on the other hand, was totally engrossed in the drama and think it may have clinched my decision to become a medical social worker. In spite of eventually changing direction, I still feel at home when visiting hospitals. At the time, I was equally attracted to a career in music and found it difficult to decide whether to satisfy the artistic or the caring side of my nature. It was a minor accident that was to influence my final decision.

The other experience marked the beginning of my life-long obsession with natural health. After suffering from measles I experienced short-sightedness and astigmatism, especially in my right eye, which I later learned indicated emotional confusion and problems with decision-making. I had discovered the Dr W.H. Bates system of improving eyesight (explained in his book *Better Sight without Glasses*) and persuaded my parents to let me undergo the treatment. My mother was very sceptical, but this spurred me on even more. My father met me in London and took me to the Harley Street practice of two sisters, the Miss Scarletts, who worked as a team.

Eye exercises that awakened my interest in natural health

The eye exercises that helped to cure my short sight and astigmatism are outlined below. They combine relaxing and exercising the eye muscles adequately whilst avoiding eye strain.

Splashing

Purpose: To stimulate and soothe nerves and muscles and cleanse the eye of impurities.

Method: Morning – flick warm water against the eyes (eyes should be open) and follow with cool water to stimulate. Evening – commence with cool water then soothe with warm water.

Repetitions: Repeat both morning and evening for a few seconds until desired result is felt.

Palming

Purpose: Improves vision by releasing tension in the optic nerve, relaxes tired muscles and increases the supply of nutrients and the removal of waste products as a result of warmth from the hands that draws more blood to the area. Will also help to prevent headaches.

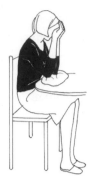

Method: Sit comfortably, elbows bent and resting on a cushion (or similar) on a table. Place 'heels' of hands on the cheek bones and cover the eyes lightly with the palms. If images or spots pass in front of the eyes, just accept them and relax. (Imagine serene pictures of the sea or countryside if this helps to induce a feeling of relaxation, but this is not necessary.)

Repetitions: 5 to 10 minutes, twice daily.

Pendulum swing

Purpose: To enable eye muscles to be exercised comfortably to their limit in all directions.

Method: Sit comfortably. Without moving the head, swing eyes from left to right as far as possible, then up and down. Next combine the two movements by describing an upward half circle to the right followed by a downward half circle, to and fro. Repeat to the left.

Repetitions: Approximately 10 of each.

Eye circling

Purpose: To increase the range of the eye muscles, particularly at the sides.

Method: Sit comfortably. Move the eyes slowly as if looking at a large clock, pausing for a second at each hour. Blink and return in an anticlockwise motion. The head should **not** move, only the eyes, and make sure they describe as large a circle as possible. Concentrate especially at the three o'clock and nine o'clock positions where the eye muscles are laziest.

If one eye is weaker than the other, use an eye patch and exercise the weak eye twice as often as the stronger one. To improve nerve and muscular co-ordination, speed up the movement and dart the eyes quickly from the numbers to the

centre of the clock and on to the next number; alternately, all
the way round and back again.

Repetitions: At least 3 times.

Focusing

Purpose: To increase the ability of the eyes to focus near and far with
equal clarity.

Method: Sit comfortably. Hold a finger about 6 inches in front of the
nose. Look deliberately at the tip of the finger, then at some
object at least 20 feet/6 metres away, noting any difficulty in
either object coming into clear focus. Blink and repeat.

Repetitions: 10.

Progressions: Try to focus on objects at different distances in quick
succession, some in the light and some in comparative
darkness.

There is no doubt that blurred vision can often occur when
eye muscles are tired and tense. In addition to the eye
exercises, a novel way to improve your focusing and exercise
muscles with ease is to wear a pair of 'pin hole' glasses for
a short period each day. Introduced in the last few years and
looking rather like sunglasses, they are said to improve vision
naturally through the use of scientifically designed and spaced
'pin dot' openings that change the way that light enters the
eye. I, myself, have used them and found that small print
becomes clearer and sharper. To begin with the glasses should
be worn for just a few minutes daily (gradually extending
the time period) while reading, watching television or using
computers. Since the glasses should be worn directly over
the eyes (not over glasses or contact lenses), if your normal
vision is poor please gain your doctor's permission before
using them.

Sitting within 6 feet/1.83 metres of a TV or any form of digital
monitor stresses the eyes and increases general tiredness.

Sunning

Purpose: To allow the eyes to absorb the beneficial sun rays.

Method: Allow the indirect rays (those before 11 am and after 3 pm) to beat on the eyelids (not the eyeballs) for a few seconds at a time.

Warning: Strong sunlight, if allowed to penetrate the eyes, can be damaging, just as it is to the skin; never look directly at the sun.

At this time I had passed my school exams and was concentrating mainly on studying for my L.R.A.M. as an external student of the Royal Academy of Music. This meant I could dispense with my glasses, a necessary part of the treatment. I practised the exercises at every opportunity and remember using the time spent in chapel services both at home and school to work with the numbers on the hymn board. Much to my mother's surprise the treatment was a total success and to this day my right eye is still strong, but my left eye has difficulty in focusing. Perhaps my left-sided energies (artistic, reflective, creative) have not been working properly. The nerves from the brain cross to the opposite side just above the eyes so that what we know as the activities associated with the right side of the brain actually travel down the left side of the body and vice versa. Just before I was to take my final practical piano exam I was stupid enough to practise a handstand and fall awkwardly spraining my wrist with the result that I stumbled in one of the piano pieces and failed by one mark. I was disappointed, but had been warned that to pass L.R.A.M. as an external student you had to be exceptionally good, and I was only ever adequate at best. Anyway, it was probably a sign that my choice of sociology for a career was the right one. The course was for those aged 19 and over so I still had a year to wait and spent it teaching piano and theory to boys at a local boarding school in the village, which I thoroughly enjoyed.

A cautionary tale: I once had perfect pitch (that is, I could recognise the aural notes played or the key the work was in), my one talent, but over the years, due to lack of use, I've lost it. Beware; what you don't use, you lose.

Lessons learned from my parents

I am pausing at this point in my story to try and identify the lessons I have learned from my parents' successes and failures and how these lessons influenced my life choices. From my mother I learned the importance of persistence and hard work in order to achieve an objective, which she demonstrated in every area of her life: in the home, in business, with her musical commitments and other pursuits. In my early years her constant encouragement stimulated me to pass all the piano grade exams and to enjoy singing in several choirs. I think her playing the organ initially attracted me to what became one of my favourite instruments, which I also learned to play in my last years at school. Nowadays I live close enough to the Royal Albert Hall to be inspired by the magnificent organ with its nine thousand, nine hundred and ninety-nine pipes, restored to its former brilliance in the early 2000s.

As my mother and I shared a similar temperament, we constantly mirrored each other's emotional states until I realised what was happening and learned to deal with the situation more logically. Her skill in training members of the Women's Institute Choir may have influenced my eventual decision to accept the challenge to teach students at the London College of Fashion.

I also think her versatility and ingenuity in co-producing the W.I. scrap book, writing other booklets and, most of all, the founding of the Perigoe Workshop Museum inspired me to pursue my own individual interests and write my self-work manuals.

On the other hand, I think I subconsciously interpreted her tendency to bouts of silent moodiness as being my fault, although I never understood the real reason for them. I think this had an inhibiting effect on my self-confidence; her occasional emotional outbursts frightened me into a tendency to seek peace at any price and suppress my feelings. My mother's gaucheness in social situations resonated with my own shyness, yet at the same time I was able to use the example of my father's easy social manners to work at overcoming my shyness.

From my father I learned what it meant to be a good citizen. He was very patriotic which he demonstrated by flying the flag (literally) on suitable occasions and standing to attention whenever the National Anthem was played, even when it was played on the radio. He was always stirred by the music of brass bands. I associate these aspects of my father with his stability and sense of tradition. I believe the combined influence of his patriotism, Christian beliefs and the generation into which he was born, (1893), has enabled me to appreciate the unifying effect of good tradition and balance it against my need for independent thinking.

I also admired the fact that in spite of a stutter my father became a Methodist local preacher and took up other posts in the community that involved public speaking. I think this influenced my decision to overcome my own fear and accept the challenge to speak from the pulpit of the City Temple in the early 1950s. My father often used his ability to act as a mediator in difficult situations, which I also have been able to do. But although he had more finesse than my mother, it often required her insistence for him to muster sufficient determination (or courage) to confront and deal with a problematic situation firmly, as I myself had to do in adult life.

Both my parents were keen for me to find fulfilment and my father harboured hopes that I would become a doctor. As I was never sufficiently good with science subjects, becoming a doctor was out of the question. But my father's hopes may have influenced my decision to become a medical social worker. Although he never lived to witness my spiritual journey and eventual metamorphosis as a natural health therapist, I hope he would have understood and approved my choice.

College years: 1946–1949

I moved to London in the autumn of 1946 prior to studying Sociology at Bedford College (part of London University) in Regents Park. On my course I met girls who had served in the armed forces, some of whom remained life-long friends. At the same time, their experience only served to emphasise my sense of immaturity as did the practical work with East Enders, living in tenement buildings, and working in a residential children's home ... and so on. I found the syllabus interesting and well constructed. It covered such subjects as the Machinery of Government, Social Administration, Ethics, Psychology, Physiology, and the Law. We also examined the Beveridge Report which formed the basis of the National Health Service (NHS) and social security systems that were implemented by the post-war Labour Government and became today's welfare state. Sir William Beveridge (a Liberal) believed that everyone should be taught the elements of health so that eventually the health of the nation would improve and the NHS would cost less. Equally, he considered that the benefit systems would act as a temporary bridge to help people until they could get on their feet again. He never intended the system to undermine self-reliance. At the time, no one could have foreseen the speed at which the genie came out of the bottle. The fact that for the first time everyone could have free false teeth and glasses and get treatment for any condition led to unimagined demands that have continued to increase over subsequent decades.

Today we have a burgeoning benefit culture and an NHS which resembles an over burdened juggernaut slowly grinding to a halt. In my view, the NHS has very little to do with real health, commendable though the system may be. It concentrates almost exclusively on prescribing ever more complex pharmaceutical drugs, all of which have possible side-effects, and/or using increasingly spectacular surgical techniques. Both methods can extend the lives of patients by removing the signs of disease, but do little to deal with the inherent causes, which in the long term lead to an increase in chronic diseases. I think it would be better renamed The National Disease Service! Ironically, a health centre was opened in Peckham in the early post-war years for the purpose of teaching the principles of health and prevention of disease, but closed some years later due to lack of interest. In these days, early diagnosis has become confused with prevention and few people seem to have noticed the difference.

To continue with my story, while at college I remember being given a day's holiday to celebrate the wedding of Princess Elizabeth (later the Queen) and Prince Philip. It was a rainy November day in 1947, but seeing the happy couple travelling down the Mall en route to their honeymoon was an uplifting spectacle that brightened those post-war years. Although it was a relief that the war had ended, bomb craters were still everywhere and food and clothing rationing continued for some years.

Early career as a medical social worker
1949–1957

After qualifying I specialised in medical social work with further training in various hospitals in London, Birmingham and Aberdeen, finally getting a job in Dulwich Hospital in 1949 and moving to St Bartholomew's Hospital (Barts) in 1952. It was interesting work helping patients deal with social factors that might have contributed to their illness and then assisting their recovery by organising convalescence, helping them with special diets where indicated or perhaps a home-help, change of job or improved housing conditions where appropriate. But in those days, I found it difficult to keep detached and I became too emotionally immersed in the patients' problems, feeling that I was personally responsible for them.

While at Barts I worked with several eminent surgeons. One operated on Sir Anthony Eden (Prime Minister at the time of the 1956 Suez Crisis). Sadly, Eden suffered complications and never returned to full health. Sir John Betjeman, the poet laureate, had an office nearby and was often seen walking round the wards offering cheer to the patients. The principle underlying social work was to help people to help themselves (as opposed to spoon-feeding them) and this principle has remained the basis of my work ever since. I firmly believe in the precepts so admirably described by Abraham Lincoln in 1865:

- You cannot bring about prosperity by discouraging thrift.
- You cannot help the wage earner by pulling down the wage payer.
- You cannot help the poor by destroying the rich.
- You cannot keep out of trouble by spending more than you can earn.
- You cannot build character and courage by taking away initiative and independence.
- You cannot help men permanently by doing for them what they could and should do for themselves.

Help from an invisible source

During my student years and beyond, I attended the City Temple Church (bombed in Holborn viaduct and re-housed in Marylebone Presbyterian Church, Edgware Road prior to rebuilding). The minister was the Rev. Dr Leslie D. Weatherhead who happened to be the father of a school friend. He was one of several famous preachers of the day, two others being William Sangster and Donald (later Lord) Soper. All three attracted large congregations.

I enjoyed singing in the choir and was a founder member of the youth club. This led, in 1951, to my being asked to speak from the pulpit at the annual youth service. A terrifying thought, but I felt I had to rise to the challenge. This resulted in my first experience of help from a higher source. I was in my parents' home for the weekend not having a clue what I was going to say, when, suddenly I seemed to be 'given' the words, possibly the response to my cry for help. I immediately felt uplifted into a safe place where fear did not exist. This feeling lasted during my journey to London through the service itself and beyond into the next week.

During this period I continued playing the piano regularly and enjoyed singing in the Royal Choral Society, led by Sir Malcolm Sargent, a very inspiring and charismatic conductor. Choral singing, for me, has always been an exhilarating and spiritually uplifting experience. During the performances of the Messiah, when we crescendoed to the climax of the Amen chorus I fully expected the vibrational force to literally raise the roof of the Royal Albert Hall. Sadly it never did!

A fateful relationship

At the end of 1951 I met Jack, the man who became the love of my life, though sadly we never married. From today's perspective I am beginning to understand that we may have had separate destinies to fulfil but it has taken well over 50 years of suppressed heartbreak to reach this point. We met at the City Temple Church through a fellow student at the Royal Academy schools where he was studying at the time. I clearly remember the first time we set eyes on each other. We were part of a group of young people walking down Park Lane when he came up to me and slid his finger down my spine, which, for me, was an electrifying experience. Our first date was the day King George VI died (6 February 1952). We'd planned to go to the cinema, but as a mark of respect to the late King all cinemas were closed. So, instead, I cooked supper for him at the flat that happened to be owned by Earl Winterton and which I shared with other girls. On several occasions the Earl surprised us with treats, he introduced us to his film star guests and once took us to tea on the terrace at the Houses of Parliament, both very exciting experiences for my flat mates and me at the time.

Jack and I quickly got to know each other and he came to stay in my parents' home many times where he was accepted as a member of the family. He spent a memorable Christmas with us when he presented my parents with a painting of the front of their house and gave me a painting of the back of the house showing part of the garden in springtime. Nowadays, during our occasional phone conversations, he still refers to the family home with nostalgia.

During the late summer of 1952, we spent an idyllic holiday in Cornwall which caused great concern to my parents as they presumed wrongly that we'd been sleeping together. In those days 'well brought up' young people did not have sex before marriage. At the same time, Jack and I realised our relationship couldn't continue as it was, indefinitely. We briefly discussed getting married right away, but the timing did not seem right in view of the fact that he still had several more years of study ahead and would also have to do his National Service (all young men had to serve in one of the services in those days.) After much heart searching we reluctantly came to the conclusion that to interrupt his studies and do his two years National Service was the right decision in the circumstances.

My parents expected that we would have an 'understanding' about the future, but Jack was too young at 23 to make a commitment, some years before embarking on a career that was by no means assured of success. I was 25 at the time and already established in my career, so there was an element of imbalance and mistiming in the situation. Although we felt the wrench acutely, we continued to write regularly and meet when he had leave. One memorable occasion was watching the Queen's coronation procession from the Mall (2 June, 1953) where we had spent a cold, damp night along with the many others.

Nowadays, I can appreciate how difficult it must have been for a young artist with an all-consuming ambition to commit to an intended permanent relationship. But in those days, without any assurance of a future together and with most of my friends marrying and fully expecting I would do the same, I must have felt emotionally insecure. I was aware that I was subconsciously transferring my tension onto him and so eventually, rightly or wrongly, I made what may have been a disastrous decision, that we should discontinue writing until he'd finished his National Service and returned from his planned visit to see his father and step-mother who had emigrated to Bulawayo, at that time in Southern Rhodesia (now Zimbabwe).

The effect upon me was catastrophic. Tears flowed without warning, but especially when anyone mentioned Jack's name. I was distraught and couldn't put into words what I was feeling without bursting into tears, so I tended to bottle things up. My parents would have been worried had they known the extent of my suffering. I carried on with life, existing like an automaton. In retrospect, I think I was overwhelmed by the most intense feeling of loss I've ever experienced. With Jack I had known a closeness and a feeling of being understood that I had craved from my mother, but had never experienced because of our often tense relationship. At the time I was never sufficiently aware of how these largely subconscious issues with my mother and parting from Jack had made me emotionally vulnerable. I think this is why I was eventually drawn into another relationship that lasted more than 12 turbulent years.

After a year or so the pain eased slightly. I had become friendly with a young couple at the church, Dina and Dennis. I was fond of them both, but unbeknown to me at the time, their marriage was in difficulty and Dennis was becoming increasingly obsessed with me. My mind was on the artist and I did not realise the extent of the situation that was developing. Later on the couple's marriage broke up and they eventually divorced. The church members were convinced he and I had committed adultery, which was not the case, although I accepted that my presence had unwittingly played a part. (Years later the ex-wife who by then had happily re-married, thanked me for 'helping' her.) The minister, always a dramatic preacher, spun round in the pulpit during a sermon, pointed a finger at me (sitting with other choir members) and spoke forcefully about those who deliberately break up other people's marriages. I felt very isolated. Nonetheless, I did feel some responsibility for the situation as I knew the man was genuinely fond of me and had done a lot to boost my dented morale. Though not a substitute for love, the common interests we shared seemed a sufficient basis for a friendship. Around this period, autumn 1956, Jack re-entered my life, albeit briefly. The incident occurred when I was visiting a friend in Welwyn Garden City. The friend and I had gone for a walk and when we returned the baby-sitter said a young man had called and in that moment I 'knew' that this was Jack. Later in the evening he returned and we met for the first time in two-and-a-half years. He had come to ask for my address. Little did he know he was going to meet me. I was on cloud nine. He wanted to accompany me home, but didn't because Dennis was meeting me at the station.

The next day Jack came to Barts with a huge bunch of pink roses, but due perhaps to the influence of Dennis (he was jealous of my feelings for Jack) maybe I did not place as much significance on these roses as I should have done. Who knows? The artist then did two things, disarmingly typical of him, which confirmed he had my best interests at heart. He stood behind me at my desk and gently pulled my sloping shoulders back. After lunch he led me to the weighing scales and said very sweetly, 'Don't you think you should lose a little weight?' During his absence I had become well covered, but his gentle touch was all I needed to take immediate action. I lost the weight (from 132 pounds to 105 pounds) and improved my posture, but sadly we were not to meet again for several years.

Jack indicated he would like to continue our friendship, but Dennis managed to convince me that I owed him loyalty and should not continue to meet Jack. So I reluctantly told him it would not be wise to see him for the time being and the following year he moved to Canada to follow his career.

Emotional insecurity
and a co-dependent relationship

A few years later Dennis's divorce was finalised and we spent more time together. My compassion for his difficult family life led to the relationship becoming stronger. I have decided to describe this relationship in some detail because it provided me with the biggest learning curve of my life and may serve to illustrate that it is possible to learn from our mistakes so that history does not need to repeat itself. Apart from learning to understand myself I learned volumes about human nature in general, which developed into a lifelong fascination with the vagaries of human behaviour that held me in good stead for the future.

There were similarities in our background in that his family were strong Methodists and several relatives had been ministers. On the other hand his father had been a manager in the local coal mine. His mother exerted a confusing and possessive influence over him and she talked openly of having married beneath herself. When he was a young boy, his mother had expected him to behave beyond his years (to compensate for what she believed to be the inadequacy of her husband) and when he grew up she undermined his confidence in order to keep him close to her. As a young boy he also had to witness the antics of an alcoholic uncle, a well respected scientist, who lived with them, but whose deceitful behaviour wreaked havoc in the family home. His mother's frantic attempts to hide the problem from the neighbours and maintain a semblance of order probably contributed to Dennis's difficulty in making decisions and his tendency to deny his problems by behaving like a control freak. This background must have made it almost impossible for him to develop his innate abilities with any confidence. He had spent time in a repertory company (which indulged his make-believe lifestyle) and he had been considered for the Methodist ministry for which he had the talents, but in my opinion would have first had to undergo psychotherapy. As it happened, he had settled into a succession of boring clerical jobs that gave him no satisfaction. It was only in his various hobbies that he enjoyed any sense of fulfilment. Dennis and I both enjoyed classical music, books, theatre and foreign travel. We travelled widely, being some of the first Westerners to visit most of Eastern Europe, including Russia, in addition to Western Europe and the United States, but soon the relationship subtly changed. Having recognised my vulnerability and helped to build up my confidence, he soon began criticising me and used emotional blackmail to increase my dependence on him. In time I realised that his criticisms were exaggerated and the relationship was descending into one of co-dependency. More is understood about these unbalanced relationships nowadays, and in my future work I was able to recognise such tendencies when helping clients in problematic relationships.

I also found that when I was discussing life's problems with college students whom I was teaching a few years later, they often told me that sharing some of my experiences helped them clarify and move on with their own problems.

Unbalanced relationships

These relationships, which may be close ones of marriage, are based on the precarious balance of each other's weaknesses and strengths and usually break down when one or other learns to become more self-reliant. It is very rare that the two people 'grow' at the same rate. One partner may try to transfer a personal fear onto the other, which may take the form of a verbal or even physical attack. The recipient may attract this situation if it happens to mirror a subconscious fear of his/her own. If the recipient is honest, he/she will recognise the element of truth in the verbal accusation made by the partner and work to overcome the particular fault. Then it will be easier to project a mental atmosphere of goodwill. As well as dispersing any vestige of compensating fear, this actually creates a 'barrier' through which the violence does not penetrate, which I was to discover for myself later in the relationship with Dennis. Such relationships are unbalanced and contrary to the Law of Harmony where opposites are attracted to each other to form a harmonious balance. They should not be confused with more normal relationships where each partner simply complements or enhances the other and each is given the loving atmosphere and freedom in which to express his/her best self.

Happiness, which many people seek as a primary aim, is a by-product. It is only by working with the conditions confronting us, building something creative out of discontent, enjoying to the full all that is good and sharing it with others that we find happiness. A few years later I studied spiritual psychotherapy and learned of the stages of development from instinctive to spiritual levels and the ages at which they occur.

If an individual fails to work through his/her problems at any one level during the usual time phase, then the difficulties multiply in the next time phase, so much so that further development may cease altogether. A fairly common example is that of the weak son with a domineering possessive mother, who, instead of growing up, subconsciously chooses a motherly wife. Not only is this type of man unable to cope adequately with the responsibilities of marriage and parenthood, but the problems with his own mother remain unresolved, adding further complications. An ill-equipped person such as this (equally applicable to a woman who has married a father figure) may drown his/her sorrows in heavy drinking or extra-marital affairs, and unless the partner remains content to play the parent role at the risk of curtailing his/her own development, this pattern of behaviour is likely to precipitate the end of the marriage. In such instances, where both partners are more or less equally at fault, this is a good example of unbalanced relationships, sometimes described as the 'Leaning Tower of Pisa' or co-dependent relationships.

Stages of development

Energy levels and their areas of operation	Period of optimum development
Instinctive, mechanical Unconscious reflexes; hunger.	Blueprint complete at birth.
Emotional Associated with the glands, interest in the opposite sex, formation of affectionate relationships, ability to procreate; the use of the imagination in creative expression (art, music, dancing and so on).	Puberty, teens.
Intellectual Aspiration, the development of personality and mental attributes by studying new skills, exploring new ideas, building a career, home and family.	Late teens and twenties.
Mental objectivity Beyond the ego and personality; the ability to think independently of established authority; belief in abstract ideals; awareness of and insight into individuality of self; reassessment of ability to adopt objective attitudes towards personal goals and achievements; ability to take responsibility for self-development rather than remaining a product of parental, environmental or other influences.	Thirties to early forties.
Psychic Awareness and constructive application of extra-sensory perception (intuition, telepathy and so on).	Thirties to early forties.
Spiritual Awakening to the deeper meaning of life resulting in a more satisfying philosophy; progressive enlightenment concerning the mysteries of life.	Late forties onwards.

These energies radiate as vibrations, known as the Aura, and are seen or felt by sensitives. Each area is subject to its own pattern of operation, but is strongly influenced by the state above, which is on a higher vibration. When these energy levels are correctly used, an artist, for instance, can apply his intellect along with inspiration and imagination so that the emotion can be expressed in a concrete form such as a painting or sculpture. If, on the other hand, the state below tries to over-rule the one above, an imbalance occurs. This can happen when an abstract ideal is misinterpreted by those with bigoted, less evolved minds and is seen in fanatical individuals, organisations and political dictatorships.

Knowledge of these subtle energy levels is undoubtedly useful in life. To take a personal example, I suddenly found I could get angry without losing emotional control. Faith in my ideals enabled me to direct my reasoning power with forcefulness. This knowledge also explains the havoc that is sometimes created by those with insufficiently awakened spiritual bodies who use esoteric truths and New Age therapy techniques simply as an intellectual skill for their own glorification. Their patients can be helped temporarily, but are often made to feel dependent on the healer or organisation. Those with emotional problems are often relieved by releasing old tensions and memories, but are not always given sufficient guidance as to how to put themselves together again. Similarly, those who misuse psychic powers, either innocently or deliberately, not recognising they are not identical with higher spiritual influences, can unbalance themselves and others weak enough to be influenced. This is an example of those who think the power or energies of healing are their own. They need to realise that they are merely the channel and that the continuous flow and quality of these energies is dependent upon their linking to the source.

How I lost weight
and began a course of self-improvement

To return to my weight loss, I formulated a system originally developed by an American authority that I continued to use with subsequent clients with great success.

Ideal weight according to height and frame size

A quick idea of our own 'ideal' can be based on the assumption that the correct weight for medium bone structure at a height of 5 feet should be 100 pounds and then add 5 pounds for every inch above this for women and 6 pounds for men. Deduct 5 or 6 pounds from this total if small boned. Add 5 or 6 pounds if large boned.

In 1960, the US Metropolitan Life Insurance Company produced an ideal 'weight table', that is, one that considered the weight at which good health is likely to be maintained. Even though such tables have been modified over the years, I still find this one extremely useful because it allows for the variables with regard to the lengths of limbs in relation to the trunk and for the fact that, although the measurements may be smaller, firm muscle (which one wants to have) weighs more than flabby muscle. This chart also enables those who are very overweight to aim first at the top end of the range. This gives time for the body to adjust and the muscles time to develop better tone from exercise before you decide if it is truly necessary to lose any more. Weight is usually taken wearing indoor clothes without shoes.

In today's world, with more people finding it difficult to maintain a healthy weight, some of my current clients dismiss these weight tables as unrealistic, but I still regard them as my yardstick.

Women 20 years and over

Height			Small frame		Medium frame		Large frame	
ft	ins	cm	lb	kg	lb	kg	lb	kg
4	10	147.3	92–98	41.7–44.5	96–107	43.5–48.5	104–119	47.2–54.0
4	11	149.9	94–101	42.6–45.8	98–110	44.5–49.9	106–122	48.1–55.3
5	0	152.4	96–104	43.5–47.2	101–113	45.8–51.3	109–125	49.4–56.7
5	1	154.9	99–107	44.9–48.5	104–116	47.2–52.6	112–128	50.8–58.1
5	2	157.5	102–110	46.3–49.9	107–119	48.5–54.0	115–131	52.2–59.4
5	3	160.0	105–113	47.6–51.3	110–122	49.9–55.3	118–134	53.5–60.8
5	4	162.6	108–116	49.0–52.6	113–126	51.3–57.2	121–138	54.9–62.6
5	5	165.1	111–119	50.3–54.0	116–130	52.6–59.0	125–142	56.7–64.4
5	6	167.6	114–123	51.7–55.8	120–135	54.4–61.2	129–146	58.5–66.2
5	7	170.2	118–127	53.5–57.6	124–139	56.2–63.0	133–150	60.3–68.0
5	8	172.7	122–131	55.3–59.4	128–143	58.1–64.9	137–154	62.1–69.9
5	9	175.3	126–135	57.2–61.2	132–147	59.9–66.7	141–158	64.0–71.7
5	10	177.8	130–140	59.0–63.5	136–151	61.7–68.5	145–163	65.8–73.9
5	11	180.3	134–144	60.8–65.3	140–155	63.5–70.3	149–168	67.6–76.2
6	0	182.9	138–148	62.6–67.1	144–159	65.3–72.1	153–173	69.4–78.5

Assessment of bone structure for women using wrist measurement in relation to height (in feet, inches and centimetres)

Height	Small	Medium	Large
ft: 4,11–5,2 cm: 149.9–157.5	inches: under 5½ cm: under 14	inches: 5½–5¾ cm: 14–14.5	inches: 5¾–6¼ cm: 14.5–16
ft: 5,2–5,4 cm:157.5–162.6	inches: 5½–6 cm: 14–15	inches: 5¾–6¼ cm: 14.5–16	inches: 6¼–6½ cm:16–16.5
ft: 5,4–5,11+ cm: 162.6–180.3	inches: 6–6¼ cm: 15–16	inches: 6¼–6½ cm: 16–16.5	inches: over 6½ cm: over 16.5

Men 20 years and over

Height			Small frame		Medium frame		Large frame	
ft	ins	cm	lb	kg	lb	kg	lb	kg
5	2	157.5	112–120	50.8–54.4	118–129	53.5–58.5	126–141	57.2–64.0
5	3	160.0	115–123	52.2–55.8	121–133	54.9–60.3	129–144	58.5–65.3
5	4	162.6	118–129	53.5–57.2	124–136	56.2–61.7	132–148	59.9–67.1
5	5	165.1	121–129	54.9–58.5	127–139	57.6–63.0	135–152	61.2–68.9
5	6	167.6	124–133	56.2–60.3	130–143	59.0–64.9	138–156	62.6–70.8
5	7	170.2	128–137	58.1–62.1	134–147	60.8–66.7	142–161	64.6–73.0
5	8	172.7	132–141	59.9–64.0	138–152	62.6–68.9	147–166	66.7–75.3
5	9	175.3	136–145	61.7–65.8	142–156	64.4–70.8	151–170	68.5–77.1
5	10	177.8	140–150	63.5–68.0	146–160	66.2–72.6	155–174	70.3–78.9
5	11	180.3	144–154	65.3–69.9	150–165	68.0–74.8	159–179	72.1–81.2
6	0	182.9	148–158	67.1–71.7	154–170	69.9–77.1	164–184	74.4–83.5
6	1	185.4	152–162	68.9–73.5	158–175	71.7–79.4	168–189	76.2–85.7
6	2	188.0	156–167	70.8–75.7	162–180	73.5–81.6	173–194	78.5–88.0
6	3	190.5	160–171	72.6–77.6	167–185	75.7–83.5	178–199	80.7–90.3
6	4	193.0	164–175	74.4–79.4	172–190	78.1–86.2	182–204	82.7–92.5

Assessment of bone structure for men using wrist measurement in relation to height (in feet, inches and cm)

Height	Small	Medium	Large
ft: 5,6–5,8 cm: 167.6 –172.7	inches: under 5¾ cm: under 14.5	inches: 5¾–6¾ cm: 14.5–17	inches: 6¾–7½ cm: 17 –19
ft: 5,8–5,10 cm: 172.7–177.8	inches:5¾–6 cm: 14.5–15	inches: 6¾–7 cm: 17–18	inches: 7½–7¾ cm: 19–19.5
ft: 5,10–6 cm: 177.8–182.9	inches: 6–6½ cm: 15–16.5	inches: 7–7¼ cm: 18–18.5	inches: 7¾–8 cm: 19.5–20
ft: over 6 cm: over 182.9	inches: 6½–6¾ cm: 16.5–17	inches: 7¼–7½ cm: 18.5–19	inches: over 8 cm: over 20

Body mass index

Nowadays frame size is largely ignored as an indicator of healthy weight. Instead the Body Mass Index (BMI) has been used to assess body weight and classify obesity according to severity, though neither the BMI nor the weight tables can accurately assess the actual level of body fat.

Our BMI is calculated by our weight in kilograms divided by our height squared. For example:

$$\frac{\text{Weight 49 kilograms}}{\text{Height 1.52 x 1.52 metres}} = 21$$

A normal BMI is in the range of 18.5–24.9; a BMI of 25.0–29.9 is considered overweight, and a BMI of more than 30, obese.

However, recent medical studies carried out by Dr Margaret Ashwell in conjunction with Oxford Brookes University point out that as the BMI fails to distinguish between muscle and body fat, and fat around the waist is considered to be potentially harmful to the vital organs in the abdominal area, a better predictor of health would be to use the waist measurement in relation to height. It is recommended that the waist should measure less than half that of the height. For example, someone of 5 ft. 4 in. (162.6 cm) should have a waist measurement below 32 inches (81.3 cm). A more detailed assessment would be to divide the waist measurement by the height. A result of 0.4–0.5 is considered to be within the healthy range, whilst below 0.4 is classed as underweight and above 0.6 as dangerously overweight.

Calculating calorie requirements

It has been established that on average a reasonably active individual uses up to 15 calories of energy to maintain each pound of body weight each day (33 calories to maintain one kilo). An inactive person (someone who mostly lies or sits down) uses 13 calories per pound (29 per kilo) and the very active person 20 calories (43 per kilo).

In order to lose one pound we must consume 3500 fewer calories than are expended in maintaining our given weight. Therefore, if you weigh 140 pounds (lb) and are medium active, you will maintain that weight by eating and drinking 140 lb x 15 = 2100 calories a day. In order to lose an average of one pound a week you need 140 lb x 15 – 500 = 1600 daily. This is calculated on the basis of dividing the 3500 into 7 days. However assuming your desired weight is actually 130 lb you will lose weight more quickly by calculating from the desired rather than the actual weight: 130 lb x 15 – 500. When you have reached your target, maintain it with 130 lb x 15. A regular diet of fewer than 1200 calories, that is for longer than two weeks, can slow down the metabolism, causing tiredness, and you run the risk of starving the body of essential nutrients, so if the normal calculation brings your allowance to 1000 calories or less you should keep it to 1200. The taller you are and the bigger your bones, the more you will lose per week. Doctors advise against losing more than two pounds per week after the initial period of adjustment, but another pound can be lost by sufficient exercise. However, if you have only a pound or two to lose and are in good health, you will probably suffer no ill effects if you remain on a diet of 1000 calories for a maximum of two weeks, better still on alternate weeks. Several ladies have come to me completely mystified because they have not lost weight on 800 calories only to find, to their surprise that they started to lose weight after increasing their intake to 1500.

These charts proved invaluable in my own case and when working with students and clients in the 1960s, 70s and 80s at a time when the hourglass figure was still considered the norm, long before the present day obesity crisis had taken hold. In those days I found that with sufficient motivation such as preparation for a holiday, a wedding or after a baby it was possible for most people to achieve their target within a few weeks. An individually prescribed balanced calorie controlled diet could result in a progressive weight and inch loss of approximately an inch off the waist, abdomen and hips, including half an inch from the thighs, every 10–14 days, in addition to the predictable weight loss.

If the diet is combined with an individually prescribed exercise plan followed five days a week (three days per week to maintain the result) the inch loss will be greater as will weight loss once the fact that firm muscles weigh more than fat is taken into account. This could amount to around two or three pounds in all. Calorie counting can seem onerous, but once the value of basic foods is mastered it soon becomes relatively easy to make an educated guess at the calorific value of complete meals with the help of the nutritional information on food labels. It's worth noting that the labels state that 2000 calories per day is the figure often quoted as being suitable for the average woman, but this amount would maintain a weight of approximately 135 pounds so is likely to be too much for anyone below 5 ft. 6 in. in height.

I carefully reduced my intake to approximately 1000–1250 calories per day, but made sure that I ate breakfast, lunch and supper to maintain my energy levels. For example:

A choice of diets

1000-calorie diet

Breakfast: One 140 ml/5 fl oz glass fresh unsweetened fruit juice or one piece of fresh fruit.

One egg, cooked without fat and with one slice wholegrain bread and 15 g/½ oz butter or 25 g/1 oz unsweetened muesli with 140 ml/5 fl oz milk or natural yogurt with no sugar.

One cup of tea, decaffeinated or substitute coffee or herb tea, with no sugar.

Lunch: 115 g/4 oz cottage cheese or 55 g/2 oz lean meat, or two eggs cooked without added fat (unless eaten for breakfast).

A large serving of green leafy vegetables (short-cooked) or a large green salad, one piece of fresh fruit or 55 g/2 oz stewed fruit sweetened with one small teaspoon honey (added after cooking).

Dinner: 85 g/3 oz lean meat, fish or poultry. A large serving of green leafy vegetables (short-cooked) or a large green salad.

Dessert as for lunch.

Snack: Either before bed or earlier in the day if needed, one piece of fresh fruit.

Daily

allowance: 280 ml/½ pt milk or 560 ml/1 pt skimmed milk or the equivalent of natural yogurt.

15 g/½ oz butter or olive oil.

If possible 1.5–2 L of water/juices liquid from fruit and vegetable/herb and fruit teas, (excluding teas and coffees), but at least one litre should be water (1 litre = 4 average glasses).

Sea salt, a little black pepper, herbs, lemon juice or cider vinegar for seasoning.

15 g/½ oz of olive oil or butter (from daily allowance) and lemon juice or cider vinegar with seasonings as above for salad dressings.

Season vegetables after cooking to avoid vitamin loss. NO sugar.

1250-calorie diet

Here are a few examples of how to convert the previous 1000 calorie diet into a 1250 calories-a-day diet. Add any ONE of the following:

- Two 140 ml/5 fl oz cartons of natural yogurt with 25 g/1 oz honey or 15 g/½ oz honey and one piece of fruit.
- 40 g/1½ oz Cheddar cheese and one slice wholegrain bread or two crispbreads.
- 40 g/1½ oz muesli-type cereal or a toasted oat, seeds and nut cereal, preferably an unsweetened variety, milk from daily allowance. NO added sugar.
- 55 g/2 oz before cooking, brown rice, buckwheat or millet.
- Two slices wholegrain bread with 15 g/½ oz butter or olive oil and one teaspoon honey if liked.
- 170 g/6 oz uncooked weight, new potatoes or jacket potato with 15 g/½ oz butter, olive oil or other cold-pressed vegetable oil.
- 115 g/4 oz of each of the following: carrots, turnips, swedes or parsnips, with 15 g/½ oz butter, olive oil or other cold pressed vegetable oil.
- Corn on the cob with 15 g/½ oz butter, olive oil or same as above.

Most people would probably find the following daily example a lot easier to follow:

170–225 g protein food – healthily produced eggs, fish, poultry, meat, organ meat, such as liver or kidney, cheese, nuts, seeds.

390–450 g fruit (fresh, ripe and preferably raw).

390–450 g salad and short cooked vegetables including pulses (peas, beans and lentils) weight before cooking, plus boiled or jacket potatoes in moderation.

25–40 g fats preferably olive oil or butter (or cold pressed vegetable oil).

55–85 g of wholegrains or cereal including bran, wheat germ, rice, bread and other flour products – weight before cooking in the case of rice and grains.

280 ml of milk (semi-skimmed or whole or the equivalent of yoghurt).

1.5–2 L of water/juices, liquid from fruits and vegetables, fruit teas (excluding tea and coffee) but at least one litre should be water = 4 average glasses.

The above quantities represent 1250–1500 calories approximately. If your calorie needs are greater than this you should increase these amounts proportionately, bearing in mind that the needs for protein, calcium, iron and other nutrients will vary for adolescence, also those who are pregnant or feeding a baby, recovering from an illness or are very physically active.

In addition, two nights a week I soaked in a very hot bath into which I had dissolved some mineral salts (no longer available today) similar to commercial Epsom Salts (magnesium sulphate) which had the effect of drawing out excess waste products through the pores, by means of perspiration. If you would like to try an Epsom Salts bath, here is the procedure. Dissolve 1–3 pounds in very hot water and soak yourself for 10–20 minutes, then close the pores with a cold splash. After drying thoroughly spend a restful evening and go to bed early. On a diet you always lose more the first week (because of the difference between the calories in the former eating pattern which maintain the higher weight and those in the reducing diet). But the loss will eventually settle down to one to two pounds per week, plus an extra pound from the special baths.

Motivation is the key. Initially I was shocked into my self-improvement programme by the artist's action, but I quickly realised that it would only succeed permanently if I did it for myself. My regular progress encouraged me to continue as did my increased self-confidence which provided the momentum to achieve my objective. It's important to be busy during a self-improvement programme and I chose an evening class entitled 'Poise, Dress, Personality'. In eight weeks I had lost in the region of 27 pounds and gone down two to three dress sizes. I was careful to weigh just once a week on the same scales at the same time of day and in the same clothes to avoid the confusion from natural fluctuations that can occur throughout the day.

Inspired by the 'Poise, Dress and Personality' course, I decided to have treatment for my bunions at one of the Dr. Scholl's foot clinics, which have all but disappeared today. The bunions developed originally after wearing an innocent looking pair of flat shoes which pressed on the big toe joints causing them to swell with pain. I was given a course of foot massage, foot exercises and faradism (a treatment where an electrical impulse is applied to the muscles causing them to contract involuntarily, which strengthens the foot muscles). The pain and swelling vanished permanently and because of my subsequent life in exercise my foot muscles have remained strong although my feet are still ugly. Current day bunion operations are more successful and recovery is quicker than formerly, but as I am symptom free I have not been tempted to have the operation.

Cosseting the feet
My advice for anyone who has calluses, corns, bunions or athlete's foot is to pay a visit to the chiropodist as I did.

You can also improve the appearance and comfort of feet and legs by exercising them regularly. The combination of strong foot muscles correctly used in walking and well-fitting shoes should improve matters further and remove any possibility of future calluses and corns. Shoes should be long enough for the ball of the foot to be flat. They should also fit firmly around the heels and sides of the feet to support them and the toes must be able to move freely. To test for correct balance when buying high-heeled shoes,

35

place a coin inside the shoe on the heel section; it should not move, if it does, the heel is too steep.

Most of us treat our feet like poor relations, but they should be treated like a best friend and receive at least as much care and attention as our hands. They certainly take more strain. Use a pumice stone to rub off dead, dry skin. If the skin is dry or even cracked, apply a cream twice daily and include the cuticles. If your feet perspire too much, wipe them with surgical spirit; you may also find the tissue salt Silica useful to treat a minor corn. Try to make sure the corn pad stays in place for several days; this will allow time for the root to be removed. I have managed this successfully, but chiropodists do not approve of them because of the possibility of healthy skin being damaged if the corn pad moves out of place.

Exercises for the feet, calves and ankles
Breathe rhythmically throughout.

Arching
Purpose: To strengthen muscles on the sole of the foot and prevent flat feet.

Method: Sit on a chair. Press pads of the toes against the floor, then draw up the muscles on the soles of the feet to accentuate the arches; relax. Exercise one foot at a time to begin with as one foot may be stronger than the other.

Repetitions: Approximately 5 with each foot.

Progressions: (i)   With practice, hold the contraction for 3 seconds and later on for 5 seconds.

(ii)   As for progression (i) but in a standing position.

Rolling
Purpose: To increase flexibility in the joints of the instep and tone muscles

that enable the foot to turn outwards and inwards.

Method: Sit on a chair. Roll to and fro from outer to inner borders, either both feet together or separately if one foot is stronger than the other.

Repetitions: Approximately 5 with each foot.

Progressions: (i) The same movement but in a standing position.

(ii) Try to roll further in each direction.

Toe spreading (abduction and adduction)

Purpose: To increase flexibility of the toes.

Method: Sit without socks or tights on (this exercise can also be done in the bath). Spread toes as far apart as possible; return to the starting position.

Repetitions: 5.

Progression: Try to spread toes further apart and hold the stretch for 5 seconds.

Toe flexion and extension

Purpose: To increase tone and flexibility of the toe muscles and joints.

Method: Sit and pick up a ball of cotton wool with the toes and pass it to the other foot; repeat to and fro.

Repetitions: 5.

Toe circling and pulling

Purpose: To increase flexibility of the toe joints.

Method: This exercise can be done in the bath or when drying, or when doing a pedicure. Grasp each foot in turn with the left hand and move each toe in a circle once clockwise and once anticlockwise; finally pull each toe gently.

Repetitions: 3 circles, increasing to 5 in each direction, followed by a pull.

Stretching instep

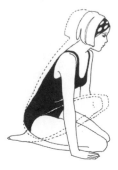

Purpose: For lengthening the muscles on top of the foot (instep).

Method: From a kneeling position, sit on the heels, place hands on the floor on the outer side of each knee, fingertips adjacent with the knees. Press down with the hands and lift the knees. Breathe in before you start and breathe out as you lift the knees.

Repetitions: 5, progressing to 10 or more, according to need.

Progressions: Lift the knees progressively higher so that only the toes remain on the floor.

Rocking from balls of feet to heels

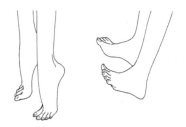

Purpose: To increase flexibility of the ankle joints and the joints at the base of the toes, also to tone muscles on the shin and the calves, and to trim the ankles.

Method: Sit on a chair. Raise the right heel, then rock back on to the heel to raise the toes, as high as possible in each direction, to and fro. Repeat with the other foot.

Repetitions: 5 with each foot.

Progressions and adaptations: If the feet are equal in strength, exercise both feet together, keeping them parallel. Increase repetitions to 10. (Lifting the heels firms the calf muscles; lifting the toes firms the shin muscles and stretches the calf muscles.) Hold contractions for 5 seconds, then relax.

To improve the shape of the calves and increase the range of muscle movement, stand with the balls of the feet either on a bottom stair or on a pile of books. If the calf muscles on the inside of the leg are too flat, exercise with the heels together and toes apart.

For practice in the bath; press the ball of the foot against the end of the bath followed by the heel; try this with just the ball of the foot if the calf muscles need tightening.

Ankle circles

Purpose: To increase flexibility of the ankle joint and improve shape.

Method: Sit, legs crossed above the knees, and with the top of the foot, describe as large a circle as possible in each direction, keeping the lower leg still. Repeat with the other foot.

Repetitions: 5, in clockwise direction followed by 5 in anticlockwise direction.

Progressions
or
alternatives: Increase repetitions to 10. 'Write' the alphabet or your name and address in capital letters with each foot in turn. (This can also be done in the bath or while watching television).

Personal crisis – my search for whole health

In 1957 my life came to a crossroads that led me to search for whole health, physical, emotional, spiritual. Factors in both my personal and professional life contributed to my eventual decision to leave Barts and completely change direction in my career. My work had become increasingly involved with terminally ill cancer patients. I was concerned by what I saw as the patronising attitudes of some social workers towards the patients and I constantly asked rhetorical questions such as 'Why can't doctors find more cures?' 'Why is there so much suffering?' and 'What is God doing about it?' My health was poor, my resistance to infection was low, I slept badly and I was constantly exhausted and suffered frequent coughs and colds. The final straw came when I succumbed to a violent infection in one of my finger nails, which I had to have removed because I failed to respond to one of the early antibiotics. The surgeon cut too deeply into the nail bed so that the new growth was permanently damaged. It happened to be the third finger on my left hand, which may or may not be significant!

In addition to my problems at work, my unhappy personal life caused my life to turn upside down and me to ask one thousand and one questions about life's apparent inequalities. All of this resulted in a pressing need to take time out to reassess my situation and find satisfying answers to the true meaning of life and health. It was a long search over many years but one that would provide opportunities for self-examination and the building of self-esteem and self-reliance. My faith in God, whatever that means, had been tested to the core, but I never lost my basic optimism and belief that good will always succeed in the end. I gradually found answers by reading everything I could find about physical and spiritual healing, often almost bursting with enthusiasm as new ideas seemed to spring out of the pages like long lost friends reminding me of forgotten truths. At the same time I was painfully aware that I would not benefit from my discoveries unless I worked on myself to understand my weaknesses and strengths, and overcome my emotional neediness.

Emotions and health

I came to a deeper understanding of the relationship between emotions and health and realised that there is no limit to the changes for the better that we can achieve.

Many of us do not realise how unfit we actually are, probably because we cannot see inside our bodies – or our minds. Our mental attitude affects our health for better or for worse every second of the day. Yet, few of us seem to recognise that tomorrow's health is determined by today's habits.

Doctors are now convinced that many more illnesses than were once thought are psychosomatic in origin. Although the effects may be seen and felt in the physical body, the roots lie in the emotions. When we respond to situations negatively, experiencing emotions such as apprehension, fear, envy, frustration or resentment, we trigger unconscious reactions in the autonomic (automatic) nervous system and in the endocrine glands. The heart rate, for instance, may speed up and the digestion slow down to help us cope with the situation. Unless we change our attitude (or solve the problem), these reactions continue indefinitely, in time upsetting the body's natural rhythm. Worse still, if we suppress our fear and anxieties instead of facing up to them, we become even less likely to stop these hidden reactions and they can eventually result in malfunction.

That this process can happen has been known for some time. What is now becoming clear is the degree to which negative emotions can be re-channelled into helping us overcome sickness and disease. If we can think ourselves into illness, then it must follow that we can think ourselves into good health.

Positive energies

To keep in a state of wholeness, health and balance, we need both to be in tune with our own energy rhythms and those in space. We need to learn to balance the different energies (physical, emotional, mental and spiritual) in our personal systems. First by taking in the energies, then by expressing them in an outward form.

Life in all its forms originates from and is sustained by this ever-flowing energy force from which we receive health, happiness, harmony, fulfilment and all good things, a continuous inflow followed by an outflow, as in breathing in and out. On a physical level, we receive this energy from sunlight, fresh unpolluted countryside, sea or mountain air, spring waters and the fruits of the earth (that is, food in a natural state, sun-ripened and uncooked, if possible). On a mental and spiritual level, we receive it from the inspiration of great music, painting, literature and drama; in the unselfish giving of our talents and in the love of our friends and family; in fact from everything that expands our capacity for living. Our choice of mental and spiritual food (books, music, art and so on) and how we express it is as important as the energy from physical food (including sunlight, fresh air and water) that needs to be channelled into physical activity, internally (as in the transportation of nutrients and waste products through the system) as well as externally in sport and other forms of exercise.

Negative energies
Misuse of energy (using it too much, too little or destructively), causes sickness, disharmony and unhappiness; all things which restrict our capacity for living a full life. The evidence is all around us in the many forms of disease, family and industrial strife, vandalism, crime, revolution and wars. Even earthquakes and volcanoes may be part of this pattern. Man's ignorance of the natural laws which govern the universe has disturbed not only the workings of his own body, but also the natural order in nature and, latterly, outer space.

When energy is used wrongly it is not always possible to detect which type of energy is being misused. This is because energies tend to interact and to some degree compensate for one another. If you skip breakfast, or are physically exhausted, it may feel like a miserable day, but the real cause can be a drop in blood sugar.

The balancing act

Good news or an unexpected loving phone call can produce a tremendous upsurge of energy, no matter what your physical condition. Mental exhaustion may disappear after a brisk walk. An emotional upset will lose its edge after digging the garden or doing some overdue chores, and a more severe shock will respond to quiet meditation and the reading of whatever religious, philosophical or literary text a person may find appropriate. In order to keep the energies flowing (and avoid the effects of misuse), we need to balance input with output; a constant challenge. On a physical level, for instance, this would result in a steady body weight.

Whether we use the energies for good or ill, they stem from the same force and Nature will find ways and means of restoring the balance. If the energies are not controlled, they threaten to destroy life, but once controlled, they can be taken into the heart as unselfish love and into the head as Divine Intelligence. But this requires a high degree of evolvement, which, apart from rare flashes of inspiration, only great teachers like Christ and the Buddhas ever attain.

Light is life; life is movement – stagnation is death

For me, this is true on every level – spiritual, mental, emotional and physical. It is true both within the human body and in the way we express ourselves in the outside world. And the principle applies equally to all forms of life whether on an individual, national, planetary or universal level.

Light, whether cosmic or solar, can be described as energy in movement. The energies given forth by the sun produce vibrations which are converted into light waves (some visible, some invisible) as they penetrate the earth's atmosphere. These light waves have different rates of vibration and are known collectively as electro-magnetic energies. Scientists now know that all matter ranging from human to so-called inanimate objects are both made of and emit these vibrations, producing an atmosphere or aura which some people are able to see in colour, but which we all feel even though we may not understand the source.

According to Albert Einstein, all matter is thought vibrating at a lower frequency. So perhaps it is not too far-fetched to think of God as having had an inspired thought which caused an outpouring of energies, which by transmutation into all the many elements, became the Universe. The universe is an ocean of movement and the motion of the earth and planets produces gravitational force which holds them suspended in space. If this movement were to stop, the earth and planets would collapse.

On a mental level we talk of 'throwing light' on a subject, of special people being a 'shining light' radiating vitality, warmth or special gifts. I think of God as the source of Spiritual Light and ourselves as radiating sparks of light. In the Bible, Christ has been described as the 'Light of the World'. On a physical level, if we do not get enough sunlight we are unable to absorb certain vitamins and minerals, our growth is stunted and we become sick. All living creatures would suffer indirectly if plants could not get enough light for their growth.

Inside our bodies cells are renewing and disintegrating continuously; oxygen is circulating through our bloodstream; food is being digested, assimilated and turned into energy; wastes are being eliminated. Everything is moving. When our hearts stop beating or we stop breathing, we die. Without mobility our joints become stiff, our muscles become flabby and waste away, and all our body processes gradually slow down. Without emotional and mental stimulation we become depressed, lethargic, dull and stupid, and our lives gradually deteriorate.

We must use energy to release more energy. From the moment of birth we are linked to the movement, rhythm and mathematics of space which gives us night and day and the seasons. We thus inherit our astrological health with tendencies in the universe as it was at the very moment of birth, the place, the time of year, the day and time of day.

We all have times of the day and seasons when we are less or more energetic. If we are in touch with these rhythms we get a 'feel for time' so that we are more likely to be in the right place at the right time.

To everything there is a season and a time to
every purpose under the Heaven: a time to be born
and a time to die; a time to plant, and a time to
pluck up that which is planted.
Ecclesiastes, *Chapter 3, Verse 1.*

There is a tide in the affairs of men,
Which, taken at the flood, leads on to fortune;
Omitted, all the voyage of their life
Is bound in shallows and in miseries.
Shakespeare, *Julius Caesar Act 4, Scene 3.*

In many ways we are the microcosm within the macrocosm. This applies as much to ourselves as to the simple atom that is linked to the solar system; as electrons circulate around its nucleus, planets circulate around the sun.

The fact that all living things are composed of the same elements helps us get our own values into perspective and to accept that we are part of a whole, whether we like it or not. It gives us a healthy respect for all nature, wind and tide, trees, flowers, insects, fish and animals. We are affected by both good and bad influences, for example, wars, earthquakes and economic slumps, as well as scientific discoveries used for the benefit of mankind, great paintings, music, poetry, literature and drama. But come what may, we remain within the protection of spiritual and natural laws which determine order in our universe and from which we cannot escape. We may get hurt or delay our progress if we break them, but the more we recognise and co-operate with them, the more we can speed our progress and the progress of those within our influence towards the realisation of our full potential.

We are all joined by an invisible thread to the unseen world through which we can draw creative thoughts and inspiration and to which we return, minus our physical body, when we 'die'. Our physical body is like a shell or sheath, our real self like a butterfly emerging from its chrysalis to fly with greater freedom in another element to see more than we ever dreamed of. And, through our invisible link, the more we work unselfishly for the benefits of others, the more spiritual knowledge and energy or healing powers will become available to us. But if we abuse them, either using them too much, too little or selfishly, then we cease to be a channel of help to other people and lose touch with the source of this special knowledge and energy.

If we embrace this stupendous conception of life, every day becomes a celebration and every moment can be savoured and lived to the full. The way we think affects every aspect of life and it is my belief that the secret of happy healthy living depends on our willingness to appreciate such things as nature's laws and the power of positive thinking.

Six keys to self-understanding

These keys represent a summary of what I came to believe at this time and used for my own development.

1. Take a long, objective look and face ourselves as we really are. This is often painful although ultimately rewarding. Learn to love and make friends with ourselves.
2. Develop the best in ourselves, including character, talents and total health and wellbeing to share with and to help others.
3. React positively, but objectively, to every situation according to our highest motives, remembering that there is always a positive side to every disaster, which will enable us to bring advantage out of disadvantage.
4. Seek greater understanding of and co-operation with natural and spiritual laws (such as gravity and cause and effect), realising that they apply equally to everyone though we are all at different stages on life's journey.
5. Accept that there are many different paths and that we have different experiences and individual lessons to learn. To judge others merely reflects our own imperfections and hinders our progress.
6. Recognise that we must take full responsibility for our development; that personal growth depends on our willingness to identify and correct any mistaken opinion, negative reaction or lack of information that may have contributed to our problems instead of placing all the blame and responsibility on circumstances or other people.

This gradual, increasing knowledge and the consequent letting go of negative thoughts makes it so much easier to cope with life. It can transform our relationships with other people, releasing the joy we all possess for truly positive living.

Ever since childhood I've been plagued by the need to understand the 'Why's of life and am aware that I irritated my mother by always demanding logical answers and never being satisfied by her emotional responses. In adult life I met with similar difficulties with vicars, colleagues and friends. Eventually I had no option but to search for answers alone, investigating other religions, visiting esoteric book shops (in particular Watkins in Cecil Court, London WC2), attending lectures from such mystics as Krishnamurti, meeting spiritual teachers at the College of Psychic Studies, (Queensberry Place, London SW7) – and finally discovering the College of Spiritual Psychotherapeutics, near Tunbridge Wells, Kent (sadly now closed) which eventually became my spiritual home. The teachings encompassed and were a 'progression' of all I had come to believe in. The Principal was Ronald Beasley, an engineer by profession, who had great spiritual insight, could see and read auras, knowing precisely what was troubling patients and was often able to heal them by the laying on of hands.

Questions to answer
before embracing a personal philosophy

Before I was able to find a stable philosophy, I found I needed to ponder certain basic issues which readers might also find helpful.

The manner in which we treat our bodies and the sort of people we become, including our appearance and degree of health and fitness, are directly influenced by what we believe life is for and the needs we wish to satisfy. Most of us in the Western world can satisfy our basic needs of warmth, food, a roof over our head, and the giving and receiving of affection. What then? Perhaps health and the ability and opportunity to express ourselves through satisfying relationships, work or hobbies, if not all three. Inevitably this leads to the fundamental questions, to which sooner or later we must seek answers:

- Who am I?
- What am I here for?
- Where have I come from?
- Where am I going?

Lord Soper, the Methodist peer, once said, 'Our practical life is nourished from within.' In other words, what makes us tick shows in everything we do: how we treat other people and ourselves, what we wear, how we furnish our homes and so on. Or, to put it another way, our thoughts are gradually manifested in our bodies and outward lives until we literally become a living image of our beliefs. Unfortunately, many of us add to our difficulties in life by becoming a hotch-potch of outworn attitudes either from our own past or of other people's beliefs, causing us to go round in circles and to be tossed about by circumstances. Or we may follow the rule book of a particular creed without real conviction and then collapse like a pack of cards in a serious crisis. Have you ever considered how you form your beliefs? Are you sufficiently motivated to read widely, study and explore every realistic avenue in your search for 'truth'? Do you examine the facts; use your reasoning powers, experience and intuition?

Are you then prepared to act upon a reasonable premise to extend your knowledge and experience?

Have you the courage to be an independent thinker or do you only 'believe' something that has been given the stamp of approval by an authority you respect or by fashionable people you wish to emulate?

The only way to establish a reliable pattern for living and solving problems is to find a stable personal philosophy strong enough to sustain us through the severest of life's crises and one that will inspire us to strive to live up to our highest ideals.

What do you believe? Do you see life as an obstacle race, a competition with your contemporaries to get ahead in your career, find friends, a husband, a wife? Is it jungle warfare, or do you think there is a niche for each one of us, a special destiny, a purpose to fulfil? Do you regard problems and difficulties as a challenge to learn? Can you turn disadvantage into advantage? Or do you think you are at the mercy of a senseless fate? Do you think that there is a reason for everything or is there a different law for some people?

Do you think the universe, as the name suggests, is essentially orderly and a unified whole? If not, what about the regularity of planetary movements, the changing seasons, the cause and effect of night and day, or the tides? Do you accept that we eventually reap what we sow, good and bad?

Surely our behaviour suggests a pattern. If we smile we know that others are more likely to behave pleasantly towards us. If we are afraid, we may act aggressively which, in turn, inclines others to do the same. If someone appears to have wronged you, can you detach yourself emotionally from the situation to examine the facts objectively, noting whether you may have contributed inadvertently to the problem? Or instead, are you more likely to react vindictively to 'pay them back' not realising that this will create a vicious circle? Have you noticed whether your reactions are based on feelings of goodwill, optimism, a sense of belonging, or unity with nature and other people? Or are your reactions mostly based on fear, especially of not being appreciated? This creates feelings of separateness, pessimism and restrictiveness, a sense of isolation, leading to attitudes of 'I can't', of 'them and us' and 'haves and have nots', even hatred, which in its extreme form can end in violence and destruction.

There is, of course, a healthy fear such as the awe we feel for God and Nature and the fear that warns us of danger. Do you recognise that love, goodwill, fear and hate are all different expressions of the same energy force?

In the current age it is all too apparent that established patterns of order and behaviour are breaking down in personal and community life. So, in order to avoid the consequences of chaos and destruction, we must grasp the opportunities to replace those patterns formerly based on rigid and prejudiced attitudes with a new order. One that combines the freedom and responsibility of self-determination with a healthy respect for all nature, also a sense of brotherhood for all mankind, regardless of race, culture, creed, and the will to live and let live.

I believe life is for abundant and victorious living. Obstacles and difficulties are no hindrance to a stimulating and joyous life; on the contrary, without them we would be less likely to discover ourselves, strive towards goals, or develop our capabilities. Needless suffering usually stems not from the events themselves, but from our failure to understand how we have contributed to the events by our attitudes or through the lack of the correct knowledge. Failures, unhappiness, unfinished projects and disastrous personal relationships all stem from misusing our creative energies. When these become blocked or stifled we suffer from 'dis-ease', if they are allowed to ebb and flow rhythmically, we are at ease with ourselves, full of joy and vitality.

Joy is a state of mind, not only dependent upon outside circumstances. It enables us to enjoy and live life expansively and express all sides of our nature. It gives us the stamina to overcome our difficulties and achieve our objectives.

Each of us is born with a quota of these energies. When they are at a low ebb, life can be reduced to an intolerable burden, or, at best, mere drudgery, whereas an abundance enables us to overcome the most impossible circumstances and climb the heights of achievement.

But the hard truth is that success in any venture, the attainment of a healthy and attractive mind and body is certainly no exception and depends upon having sufficient strength of purpose to stick to a realistic campaign long enough to obtain the desired result. As this usually involves changing certain habits for life, it is essential that we not only find a healthy eating pattern and mode of exercise we can enjoy, but a supportive practical philosophy for everyday living. The more we are inspired by a totally positive belief system, the more we are motivated to achieve and maintain our objectives. If our conviction is strong enough, we continually attract and respond to every opportunity that will enable us to fulfil the aim until we become a living manifestation of it; we become one with it. The process is the same whether the purpose is an altruistic or a selfish one, potentially helpful or harmful.

If we continue to evolve, this progressive ongoing process (in the context of health) will free us from the fetters of physical and emotional restrictiveness and open up endless expectations and horizons in other areas of life. There is no need to be deterred by the fear of added responsibilities that may result from living a busier, more fulfilled life as you will be producing more than enough mental and physical energy to deal with them. Energy is self-generating when used in a balanced way (positively and evenly), a period of activity followed by a pause. If we believe we have a soul, then the body, mind, emotions and psychic energies can become its willing instruments. Otherwise we can easily become the victim of fluctuating interests of the will, emotions, instincts and appetites, often pulling us in opposite directions. Allowing the soul to be in charge enables us to integrate all sides of our nature, to think and act decisively, freed from mental conflict and emotionally clouded vision.

Ongoing improvements to health

While I was still working at Bart's hospital, I had a period of chronic insomnia and other related problems brought on by the stress of my relationship troubles and I succumbed to taking barbiturates (strong sleeping tablets). Not only did they make me feel sick, but I must have looked ill because I remember several occasions when older people gave me their seat on the underground train. This experience, combined with my lack of response to antibiotics, gave me the impetus to find a natural cure and I subsequently found that calcium supplements and herbal tablets such as passiflora were a more effective way to address my insomnia. Another experience that helped me recognise the importance of a whole food diet was the chronic sinusitis and severe rheumatic pains I suffered at this time. In the middle of one night the sinus pain was so bad that the fear of my head bursting drove me to get out of bed, dress and walk a mile or more to St Mary's Hospital (Paddington, London). Fortunately the sight of the Casualty notice and the cold night air were sufficient to clear my sinuses instantaneously so I turned around and went straight back to bed, resolving to overcome these problems once and for all. This I did by largely giving up sugar (I had already given it up in teas and coffees when I lost the excess weight), white bread and white flour products, cutting back severely on salt, and increasing my intake of fresh fruit and vegetables. Later I was to discover that two teaspoons of cider vinegar and one teaspoon of unheated honey in water several times a day helped all the above conditions. I also discovered Biochemic Tissue Salts and found relief with Combination Q for catarrhal and sinus problems and Combination M for rheumatic pains.

Naturopaths believe that cider vinegar has therapeutic properties on account of the minerals such as calcium and potassium that it contains albeit in small amounts. They believe that when diluted in water it can promote a healthy digestion and healthy hair if used as a rinse after shampooing. When taken with honey, cider vinegar can increase the assimilation of calcium and removal of uric acid and other toxic deposits and help to relieve the symptoms of arthritis. The following is a guide to suitable dilution of cider vinegar: 1–2 tbsp of cider vinegar to 284–568 ml of water.

Biochemic tissue salts

Biochemistry is a term more commonly used to describe the chemistry of living tissue and the vital processes that occur in the body. Once an ancient Sanskrit science, it is also another natural form of healing, and was introduced in modern times over a century ago when an eminent scientist, Rudolph Virchow, discovered that every cell in the human body is composed of an infinitesimal but perfectly balanced quantity of three types of material: water, organic substances – the structural part of animal or vegetable matter (sugar, albuminous and fatty substances) – and inorganic substances (mineral salts). Although present in smaller quantities than the other two, the inorganic, or mineral elements are vital to the constant rebuilding of new cells. When there is a shortage, the body rhythm is put off balance and this gives rise to disease. A German doctor, Dr William Schuessler (1821–1881), experimented with this knowledge and formulated an abridged homoeopathic therapy, later to be taken further by Dr G.W. Carey. Still using homoeopathy's minimum doses, he worked on the basis of actually restoring balance by replacing the specific cell salts that are in short supply. In other words, biochemic therapy restores the material that is lacking, while homoeopathy uses remedies that are harmonious but not identical with the constituents of the body. Dr Schuessler's method uses twelve inorganic mineral substances, which he calls the twelve tissue salts. They are essential to life and health.

Tissue salts are subtle in their effect, quality being more important than quantity. The minute dose and the method by which they are taken (absorbed directly through the mucosal lining of the mouth), ensures complete absorption by the blood. Large doses of minerals (in their pure form without a binder such as gluconates or orotates), as for instance the iron tablets that were once prescribed for anaemia, without a suitable binder can irritate the stomach, cause constipation, and are often excreted without reaching the bloodstream. Sodium chloride in its table salt form is also too coarse for the body to absorb directly, although sodium is an essential mineral.

Functions and indications for use
I like the speedy and subtle efficiency of tissue salts and have recommended them to my clients for years. For instance, mild digestive discomfort can disappear within ten minutes and dramatic relief from severe cough and cold symptoms can be obtained within 24 hours. A number of my clients have also been completely cured of migraine headaches by regular use of these salts over a period of time.

Here is a brief summary of their functions and indications for use:
1   *Calc. Fluor.* (calcium fluoride) creates and maintains the elastic tissue of veins, arteries, skin and membranes. It preserves the enamel of teeth. A deficiency of this tissue salt gives rise to a general 'sagging feeling', to loss of elasticity, to cracks in the skin and to lack of muscular tone. Indicated in the treatment of pain in the lower back, chaps and cracks in the skin, enlarged and varicose veins, piles, prolapse of the womb, and poor circulation.
2   *Calc. Phos.* (calcium phosphate) creates and maintains bones and teeth, it has a beneficial influence on digestion and assimilation. Indicated in the treatment of lack of energy, debility, ill-nourished states, weak digestion, infants' teething troubles, chilblains, simple anaemia in conjunction with Ferr. Phos.
3   *Calc. Sulph.* (calcium sulphate) a constituent of connective tissue, skin and mucous membranes. This tissue salt promotes the elimination of non-functional organic matter so that it may not lie dormant or slowly decay and injure the surrounding tissues. Cal. Sulph. promotes healing. Indicated in the treatment of impure blood, acne, gumboils, sore lips, and wounds that are slow to heal.
4   *Ferr. Phos.* (phosphate of iron) oxygenates the blood by taking up oxygen from the air inhaled into the lungs. It gives strength and toughness to the walls of the blood vessels, especially the arteries, hence its value in the treatment of ailments associated with advancing years. It is indicated in the treatment of sore throats, coughs, colds, fevers, inflammation,

throbbing headaches. Powdered Ferr. Phos. applied externally checks the bleeding of cuts, abrasions and so on. Ferr. Phos. is the pre-eminent biochemic first aid.

5   *Kali Mur.* (potassium chloride) is a blood conditioner that unites with fibrin and works in close relation with Nat. Mur. A deficiency of Kali Mur. may be seen in the form of white or greyish fibrinous discharges and a white-coated tongue. This tissue salt helps to maintain the fluidity of the blood. It is indicated in the treatment of inflammatory conditions (in alteration with Ferr. Phos.), coughs, colds, swollen glands and chronic rheumatic swellings. It is helpful in the treatment of children's ailments.

6   *Kali Phos.* (potassium phosphate) is a constituent of nerves and brain. Indicated in the treatment of nervous disorders, including sleeplessness, depression, nervous headaches, and for skin ailments and digestive upsets associated with 'nerves'.

7   *Kali Sulph.* (potassium sulphate) acts in conjunction with Ferr. Phos. as an oxygen carrier. It has an affinity with the cells forming the lining of the skin and mucous lining of internal organs. Indicated in the treatment of skin and scalp disorders or for scaling of the skin with sticky exudations and for yellowish or greenish catarrhal discharges. It helps to condition hair and nails and is indicated when there is a feeling of stuffiness or desire for cool air. Assists in treatment of psoriasis and athlete's foot.

8   *Mag. Phos.* (magnesium phosphate) is anti-spasmodic. Indicated in the treatment of spasmodic darting pains, cramp, hiccups, fits of coughing, flatulence, neuralgia and supplements the action of Kali Phos. in conjunction with the nervous system. Mag. Phos. will usually act more rapidly if taken with a little hot water.

9   *Nat. Mur.* (sodium chloride) is a water distributor. It controls the degree of moisture within the tissues. It is indicated in the treatment of watery symptoms or for excessive dryness in any part of the body: streaming colds, headaches with constipation, difficult stools, loss of taste or smell, dryness of the skin and mucous membranes, flow of tears, wet eczema. It is also used for slow digestion owing to too little hydrochloric acid. Nat. Mur. balm, applied externally, soothes the bites and stings of insects.

10 *Nat. Phos.* (sodium phosphate) is an acid neutraliser. It is indicated in the treatment of acidity, heartburn, poor digestion, impaired assimilation, a yellow-coated tongue, rheumatic twinges, and allied conditions. It maintains the alkalinity of the blood and assists in the digestion of fatty foods.

11 *Nat. Sulph.* (sodium sulphate) eliminates excess water. Indicated in the treatment of water-logged states and associated ailments. For liverishness, bilious upsets, sick headache, influenza, and water retention.

12 *Silica* (silicic oxide) has a deep-seated action as a cleanser and eliminator. It promotes suppuration and hastens the discharge of non-functional organic matter. It restores activity of the skin in cases of checked perspiration and remedies offensive perspiration. It is also a constituent of hair and nails. This tissue salt is indicated in the treatment of boils, styes and tonsillitis, and dissolves urates lodged around joints and muscles in rheumatic conditions. It has a beneficial effect upon poor memory and absent-mindedness. It also combats brittle nails and lack-lustre hair.

Combination remedies and indications for use

These specific combinations of tissue salts can be used for combating the following complaints:

Code	Tissue Salt	Complaint
A	*Ferr. Phos., Kali Phos., Mag. Phos.*	Neuralgia, neuritis, sciatica
B	*Calc. Phos., Kali Phos., Ferr. Phos.*	General debility, nervous exhaustion and during convalescence
C	*Mag. Phos., Nat. Phos., Nat. Sulph., Silica*	Acidity, dyspepsia, heartburn
D	*Kali Mur., Kali Sulph., Calc. Sulph., Silica*	Minor skin ailments
E	*Calc. Phos., Mag. Phos., Nat. Sulph.*	Flatulence, colic, indigestion
F	*Kali Phos., Mag. Phos., Nat. Mur., Silica*	Migraine, nervous headache
G	*Calc. Fluor., Calc. Phos., Kali Phos., Nat. Mur.*	Backache, lumbago, piles

H	Mag. Phos., Nat. Mur., Silica.	Hay fever and allergic rhinitis
I	Ferr. Phos., Kali Sulph., Mag. Phos	Fibrositis, muscular pain
J	Ferr. Phos., Kali Mur., Nat. Mur.	Coughs, colds, chestiness
K	Kali Sulph., Nat. Mur., Silica	Brittle nails, falling hair
L	Calc. Fluor., Ferr.Phos., Nat. Mur.	Varicose veins and circulation
M	Nat. Phos., Nat. Sulph., Kali Mur., Calc. Phos.	Rheumatism
N	Calc. Phos., Kali Mur., Kali Phos., Mag. Phos	Menstrual pain and allied conditions
P	Calc. Fluor., Calc. Phos., Kali Phos., Mag. Phos.	Aching feet and legs, poor circulation, chilblains
Q	Ferr.Phos., Kali Mur., Kali Sulph., Nat. Mur.	Catarrh, sinus disorders
R	Calc. Fluor., Calc. Phos., Ferr. Phos., Silica	Infants' teething pains and to aid dentition
S	Kali Mur., Nat. Phos., Nat. Sulph.	Stomach upsets, biliousness, sick

All of these remedies can be obtained from health shops and larger chemists. The combination remedies are identified by their designated letter of the alphabet.

The pH factor

During this same period I also learnt the value of eating more alkaline-forming foods than acid-forming foods.

In order to maintain a correct chemical balance for our bodies, our daily diet should consist of four fifths (80 per cent) alkaline-forming foods and one fifth (20 per cent) acid-forming foods. All foods, after they have passed through each stage of digestion, are broken down into mineral salts that are either predominantly alkaline or acid. This process should not be confused with the predominant acidity or alkalinity of food **before** it is eaten. Citrus fruits, for instance, if correctly digested, break down finally into alkaline substances in the body, the exception being oranges which are imported in an unripe condition and are not broken down into alkaline in the body.

pH is the symbol for hydrogen ion concentration. On a sliding scale of 0–14, a pH of 7 is neutral. A pH of less than 7 is acid and one greater than 7 is alkaline. Normal blood has a pH of 7.4 (slightly alkaline) and skin has a pH of 5 or 6 (slightly acid).

Alkaline-forming foods (which should make up four fifths of the diet) are:
- all fresh and dried fruits with the exception of rhubarb, plums and cranberries
- vegetables
- salad vegetables
- nuts with the exception of walnuts, (and peanuts which are not true nuts)
- milk
- yogurt
- buttermilk
- soft cheese

Acid-forming foods (which should make up one fifth of the diet) are:
- alcohol
- meat (red meat in particular)
- eggs; hard cheese
- fish
- cereals, including grains and flour products (especially if they are refined)
- sugar (and everything to which it has been added, such as jam)
- tobacco
- salt
- white pepper (black pepper is less acid-forming)
- tea and coffee
- walnuts, peanuts, dried pulses and seeds
- fats (slightly acid-forming, vegetable oils less so than animal fats)

In general, the diets of most people are proportionately the wrong way round with the emphasis on acid-forming foods. If this imbalance can be corrected, overweight and other diet-related conditions can be relieved.

I also found that foods rich in B vitamins increased my mental and physical energy, which helped me cope better with my relationship problems. They particularly helped me to deal with situations that otherwise brought me to tears or made me feel irritable.

Foods rich in B vitamins include:
- wheat germ
- liver, heart, brains, kidney and other meat, poultry, fish
- cheese and eggs
- soya products
- wholegrain products
- brown rice
- broccoli, green peppers, avocados, green leafy vegetables
- nuts and seeds

As I mentioned previously, in 1957 my life came to an impasse requiring big changes and at the end of that year I left my job at Barts Hospital fully intending it to be a temporary break in social work. Little did I realise that my search for answers to life's problems would result in a sea-change in every area of my life. To begin with, I undertook a protracted course in health and beauty therapy. In order to keep body and soul together I took a variety of part-time jobs. One was at the Red Cross where I introduced skin care and make-up services to women patients in long-stay hospitals and sanatoria. Then I became a hairdressers' receptionist, and finally worked at Top Rank health clubs prior to moving on to the Elizabeth Arden Salon in Bond Street where initially I taught exercises. Later I was able to add nutritional advice, yoga and remedial massage, and remained there for nine happy years where my working life helped to offset my turbulent personal life.

A bitter-sweet encounter with Jack
In the autumn of 1958 I remember Jack, the artist, calling late one night at the bedsit house where I lived, which made it a very awkward meeting. We had to chat quickly on the stairs; the landlord would have terminated my tenancy if I had invited Jack into the room. In spite of this, the magnetism between us was as strong as ever. I desperately wanted to ask his help concerning my

relationship with Dennis, but decided it was unfair to involve him. Because of his generous financial offer some years later, I'm sure he would have helped me, but I probably had a subconscious need to work through my problems myself. When he told me about the girl he'd met in Canada, I felt my life was doomed, but had wanted some assurance that at least one of us stood a chance of happiness.

We've recently renewed telephone contact and when reminiscing he commented on my cool manner that night, so maybe we got our wires crossed because neither of us had the guts to reveal our true feelings that fateful night.

Twin souls/twin sparks

To this day I cannot totally explain my extreme reaction to the parting from my artist friend. I had thought that perhaps I had been emotionally immature at the time, which was true, but not enough to explain the intensity of my reaction as the same reaction has continued to occur after every brief meeting over the years. It follows the same pattern: I cry uncontrollably for about 48 hours and then, with great effort, manage to get my life back to some semblance of normality. It actually feels as if my soul has left my body to unite with his soul. The term soulmate is familiar to many people, but does not adequately describe my relationship. The only term that comes anywhere close enough is that of twin soul (sometimes called twin sparks). Little is understood of the concept of twin souls. Some people think it is synonymous with that of soulmate. I consider that I have known more than one soulmate which I interpret as souls with whom I have been especially close in previous lives. They are definitely separate entities whereas the experience I call that of twin soul is one that I can only describe as literally being two halves of one whole as if at the point of creation one soul or spiritual spark has been divided into two parts.

Aspects of my health and beauty classes

A s a result of my health discoveries and the poise, dress and personality course, I was eventually able to devise my own course which I introduced a few years later as health and beauty courses for the Inner London Education Authority (ILEA) evening classes. As all this occurred around the milestone of my 30th birthday, I resolved to remain youthful and fit in mind and body and delay the ageing process for as long as possible using entirely natural means while teaching others to do the same. As I continued to study health and beauty from within and without, I realised that helping others would continuously recharge my motivation and keep me on the straight and narrow as I couldn't risk not continuing to set a good example. Here are a few examples of the material I shared with my students in the ILEA classes.

Although I covered the usual aspects of poise, posture, etiquette, dress, hairstyles, weight control, skin care and make-up, I emphasised the concept of whole health and adapted the material to suit my students who were mostly busy working girls and mothers living on a tight budget. I stressed the importance of making good use of the natural elements of sunlight, water and fresh air, as well as correct posture and breathing.

Energy from natural elements

Sunlight

It is from the sun that we receive all the energies that make life possible on this planet, and our own internal energy cycles are linked with the sun, moon and planets. The saying 'early to bed, early to rise' is connected with the rhythm of the sun's magnetic rays. As the sun rises and sets, it creates an intense field of magnetic energy, the blue and violet end of the spectrum in the morning, and the orange and red in the evening.

Generally, most of us operate best by doing our hardest work between sunrise and noon then gradually slowing down during the afternoon, ready for recreation. The time between midnight and dawn, when the sun's magnetic energies are at their lowest, coincides with the time our temperature is at its lowest and when our energy is at its lowest ebb.

The action of sunlight on the skin enables the body to absorb vitamin D, which is necessary for calcium assimilation and healthy bones. In moderation, sunbathing increases the elimination of toxins through the skin but too much sun heat especially between 11 am and approximately 3 pm in the summer is harmful. Strong sun ages the skin, may be a pre-disposing factor in skin cancer, and causes valuable water-soluble vitamins and minerals to be lost through excessive perspiration. Sun-glasses should only be worn as a protection from strong glare, or when the sun is excessively hot. If the light is not excessive, a need for protection indicates a lack of vitamins A or B.

Whenever you sunbathe, protect your skin well with suitable sun cream for your skin type, and either cover your eyes or wear sun-glasses that protect your eyes sufficiently from all angles, as well as protecting the surrounding delicate skin. As a precaution against a headache or sunstroke, cover the entire head and neck areas, and during the strong midday summer sun (11 am–3 pm) stay in the shade.

Expose each side of your body for a maximum of ten minutes on the first day, increasing by no more than five minutes a day. Vitamin D can penetrate fair skin more easily than a dark skin, so to persist after achieving a mild tan will slow down the rate at which vitamin D is manufactured on the skin. Like other fat-soluble vitamins, vitamin D is absorbed in an oily medium, so don't wash off the sun cream for up to an hour after sunbathing. Take similar care even when you are not deliberately sunbathing, such as while gardening, and sitting or working out of doors. You should also take care when sightseeing on holiday, although the effect of the sun will not be so great in an upright position (except on the shoulders, which should be protected accordingly).

Sun creams and lotions contain differing strengths of the protection factor and this is indicated by numbers (the higher the number, the greater the protection), but the system is not uniform across the brands, so check the label. Choose one with a B complex vitamin, para amino benzoic acid (PABA), which lessens the damaging effects of the sun. (You can also take PABA as part of a vitamin B complex tablet). If you are fair skinned or it is your first exposure of the season to hot sun, use a sun cream with a high filter factor – also useful for specially sensitive areas such as the eyelids, nose, tops of arms and shoulders, backs of hands and legs, and soles of feet.

Always re-apply sun cream at regular intervals, according to the manufacturer's instructions and don't forget that if you are in a pool by the sea, the sun's rays will penetrate the water. At the seaside don't be misled by cool sea breezes or mist. You must still be protected or you may get severely burned. On a skiing holiday you will also need to use a high-protection sun screen because of the reflection from the snow. Don't forget the lips, unless you use an extra-creamy lipstick. Keep your eyes well protected by sun-glasses or goggles. At night apply moisturising cream generously.

If you do get sunburnt, apply cool water to the area, then dab it dry and apply a cooling lotion; natural yogurt or buttermilk both help, as does a homoeopathic burns ointment containing calendula and cantharis, available from homoeopathic chemists. Vitamin E is also effective both applied directly on the burn and taken internally (400–500 mg.).

Water
The treatment of internal or external disease by water (hydrotherapy) was practised in ancient times by the Egyptians, Greeks and Romans. Hippocrates is reputed to have recommended the use of 'sun-water' (rainwater). Rainwater contains not only solar energy, but more oxygen and nitrogen (needed for the building and repair of body cells) than tap water. Nowadays, though, it is quite likely to contain the air pollutants found in industrial and city areas.

Water taken internally

There is no longer any danger of getting dysentery from drinking tap water, but we cannot control the varying degrees of artificial chemicals added to our water. Some of these are known to be toxic and, at the very least, they may disturb the body's mineral balance. It is to be hoped that the inside of our bodies does not become as furred up as the inside of an electric kettle. There has been much controversy over the fluoridisation of water. Fluorine in small quantities from a natural source (available in tissue salt form as calcium fluoride) may help prevent the destruction of tooth enamel, but sodium fluoride, the type added to water is an industrial waste and not the same as calcium fluoride. If water is boiled before use, chemicals such as chlorine and calcium bicarbonate (which coats food and makes it less digestible, and lines saucepans with lime) will be removed in the steam. Distillation, which removes the water from the pollutants, is the most efficient method; but distilled water is devoid of natural minerals and trace elements as well as impurities. In contrast, the more commonly used water-jug filters remove the impurities from the water, but in varying degrees of efficiency, leaving the natural elements intact. Most types of filter remove chalk and chlorine effectively but are less effective at extracting nitrates and lead and have little or no effect on aluminium, fluoride and any other toxic substances that may be present in the tap water.

To treat the body hydrotherapeutically, drink a glass of hot, previously boiled water each morning; it will help remove toxins via the kidneys. Sixty per cent of our body consists of water and it is essential to the oxidisation process that carries nutrients dissolved in water to the cells and likewise carries waste products to the eliminatory organs. About 2 L./3.5 pt. are lost daily and this water must be replaced. Ample amounts of fruit and vegetables and salad in the daily diet will provide approximately 850 ml/1.5 pts. of liquid and the balance can be made up by water or fruit juices. Those lucky enough to have a natural fresh water spring in the garden should make full use of it and serve it to their family, animals and plants, drink it and wash in it. It is ideal for the skin. Natural spring waters are also bottled: Malvern, Contrexéville, Evian and Volvic are some examples. The last three named are known for their mildly diuretic effects so they are also helpful for removing waste matter that may be aggravating rheumatism, gout or arthritic conditions. All such waters contain natural minerals in varying degrees.

Sea water

This is of value internally. Analysis has shown that the human bloodstream contains identical minerals to those found in sea-water. In emergencies when no blood has been available, doctors have given patients sea-water transfusions. Arthritis and other joint troubles have also responded well to sea-water. A man crippled with arthritis at 96 actually walked again after drinking sea-water regularly. Filtered untreated sea-water has sometimes been obtainable in bottles from health shops, and it is customary to add it to ordinary drinking-water or to distilled water if this is preferred. However, great care must be taken to ensure that the sea-water has not been contaminated. It should come from the greatest possible depths and from an area at least 30 miles from the shore.

Water used externally

Baths

Seaweed extract baths

These have a similar but invigorating effect because of their iodine content. You can also increase the circulation and remove the dead skin with a loofah glove, or fairly stiff bath brush, and then rub the skin dry with a rough towel. This will help prevent or alleviate any tendency to 'goose pimples', which sometimes prevent the skin from breathing properly. Brushing the skin when it is dry with a soft bristle brush is also good for the circulation. It is important to rest for half an hour to an hour after these types of bath, as the perspiration will continue for a while. Then, preferably, spend a restful evening and go to bed early.

Mustard foot-bath

For this well tried old fashioned remedy, use one tablespoon of mustard powder with enough hot water to reach to mid-calf level. Foot-baths promote sleep, improve circulation, help to lower blood pressure and relieve early symptoms of a cold.

Also good for feet is to walk barefoot in the dew, especially on the grass or sand; it will help to remove toxins through the soles of the feet, and release static electricity from the body, calm the nerves and improve circulation in the feet.

Spa towns are renowned for their hydrotherapy treatment and many people still go there to 'take the cure'. Apart from the water that is drunk, there are many types of baths, including mud-baths, containing natural minerals. Underwater and hand massage is also practised.

Thalassotherapy (sea-water therapy)

This is practised at centres on the Britanny and South Atlantic coasts, where people with rheumatism, arthritis and metabolic disorders, or who are overweight and suffer from cellulite, derive much benefit. Treatments with cream and lotions based on micronised (finely ground) marine algae are also given and these products are available commercially from good chemists.

Fresh air and oxygen

Hippocrates is reputed to have regarded oxygen as the most important element for health, and lack of it as the physical root of all disease. Slow rhythmic diaphragmatic breathing in the fresh air increases oxygen intake, which nourishes and cleanses the system. Without oxygen, nutrients cannot be released to the cells nor waste products removed from the cells. Oxygen can increase resistance to disease, particularly in the lungs, nose and throat, as well as help to calm the nerves. None of us needs be persuaded of the benefits of breathing clean, fresh air, whether it is the sweet, gentle scents of country air, bracing seaweed-scented sea air or exhilarating mountain air. No wonder clinics and sanatoria are found in these areas, often near pine-forests that increase the oxygen content of the air.

As much as possible, avoid the exhaust fumes from taxis and buses, smoke-filled atmospheres, as well as air-conditioning. There is less oxygen in reconditioned air and this tires the brain more quickly, and increases the dark circles under the eyes. You can take an air bath in the seclusion of your home or garden whenever weather permits and wear loose clothing in warm weather so that the skin can breathe in more oxygen.

Oxygen's vital role
The energy for all body activities, whether for the muscles, nerves, body fluids or the activity within each cell, is supplied by the burning of nutrients obtained from foods. This occurs when they combine with oxygen, which is then exchanged for carbon dioxide. For this combustion to take place there must be a continuous supply of oxygen and the means to remove the carbon dioxide. The respiratory system performs this function by acting like a pair of bellows, although very small amounts of oxygen can be absorbed through the skin and from drinking-water and eating foods with a high water content.

The dangers of under- or over-exposure to certain elements

The Seasonal Affective Disorder (SAD) syndrome
Seasonal Affective Disorder (SAD) is a recognised condition directly related to the lack of light in winter. The symptoms include severe depression, extreme fatigue, increased appetite, particularly for sugary foods and carbohydrates, and weight gain during the winter months. This syndrome is more likely to occur in people with indoor lifestyles, especially those who are exposed to long hours of artificial light. Even on a grey overcast day there is more light out of doors. So, a daily walk is the first step to a cure, but spending several hours outside (which is advisable), may not be practical for everyone. In this case, those who suffer with severe symptoms can be helped by sitting for two hours at a time, two or three times each day in front of a special light-box that simulates the full daylight spectrum, and contains six full spectrum tubes of 40 watts each. Together they give 2500 lux (the equivalent of a bright Mediterranean summer day) and the intensity of light capable of relieving the symptoms after a week or two of this treatment.

Being sensible about the sun

I have previously referred to the dangers of too much sunlight. Even sun-beds that are reputed to have the harmful UV rays removed should, I believe, be used cautiously. Ill-effects from too much sun may not show up in the skin immediately. However, long-term exposure will encourage the skin to shrivel and tend to become leathery (depending on its type). Pigmented spots also tend to increase and any raised ones should be watched with care and medical advice sought if necessary. The sun is also known to decrease the production of collagen. Dark skins and Mediterranean skin types have more oil and natural pigment, which gives them better protection from the sun's harmful rays. In fairer skins, sufficient vitamin D has usually been absorbed with the summer's initial light tan and as long as sun oil is left on afterwards for half to one hour, complete absorption will be ensured. It is sunlight we need not sun 'heat' and we should never lie in the midday sun (between the hours of 11 am and 3 pm) in the summer months.

Posture and breathing

Efficient posture and breathing are fundamental to both physical and mental health, so body improvements should start by making any necessary improvements in our posture and breathing habits otherwise a diet and general exercise programme will be less effective. If posture is wrong, for instance, it will not be possible to perform the exercises correctly and may cause strain; if breathing is shallow there may be insufficient oxygen to ensure complete digestion of the food we eat.

Posture and breathing are interrelated. If we stoop or have very round shoulders we will almost certainly breathe shallowly as the lungs cannot expand fully in that position. Similarly, if breathing is habitually shallow, we are more likely to develop a slumped posture. Oxygen is more essential even than water or food. The body can live for hours without water, days without food but only seconds without oxygen. Lack of oxygen and failure to expel carbon dioxide from the base of the lungs will sooner or later result in poorer health. Apart from being less attractive, a slumped posture is tiring and if uncorrected can result in unnecessary depression, muscular tension, backache and joint strain.

Maintaining perfect posture

Gravity, the force that draws all objects towards the earth, affects us all the time. Having forgotten our struggles to resist it when learning to walk, we usually only become aware of gravity when we lose our balance and fall over, or when we suffer discomfort from the uneven distribution of weight either of our own body or an object we are holding. What we feel as 'weight' is actually the force of gravity and by making careful adjustments to our posture, it is possible to prevent unnecessary tiredness and wear and tear in both muscles and joints.

If we have had the benefit of a healthy active childhood, the muscles that work statically to maintain correct balance (mainly those in the back of the neck, the back and legs) will have sufficient strength to maintain our body in an upright posture. In addition, there is a complex interplay between the muscles involved in movement and nerves in muscles, joints, ears, eyes and skin known as postural reflexes. These nerves receive stimuli and convey them to different parts of the brain, which then 'confer' and send appropriate instructions to the muscles involved so that correct adjustments are made. Some of these reflexes are inborn but others are developed as the result of constant repetition and are then 'filed' in the brain as automatic patterns so that we are no longer conscious of them.

It is possible to maintain an erect posture without strain on the joints or uneven development of the muscles as long as the major joints remain in the same vertical plane, one on top of another rather like the floors of a house. In the absence of any skeletal abnormality it is possible, when in the standing position, for the line of gravity to fall through the top of the head, the mid-cervical (neck) vertebrae, the front of the thoracic vertebrae, the mid-lumbar vertebrae, the second sacral vertebra (centre of gravity), through or slightly in front of the knees and slightly in front of the ankles to a point between the feet adjacent to the instep. The weight of the body should be evenly balanced to maintain efficient posture with maximum efficiency and the minimum of effort. Energy used economically, will increase our sense of physical and mental wellbeing.

When we are tired or depressed, when we lift or carry things carelessly, we tend to slump. If allowed to continue, bad posture will eventually strain the joints and tendons that join muscles to joints.

To correct faults, we must become conscious of sensations indicative of incorrect posture such as tight muscles, discomfort, pain or uneven weight distribution and take counter-action before the habit becomes established and damage is done.

Once structural changes have occurred in joints and bones these are difficult, if not impossible, to cure but they can be prevented with gentle persistence and comparatively little effort. You can also take heart from the fact that good posture and breathing can improve your shape which, combined with a light step and a smile, not only makes you feel better – because you look better, and because good posture uses less energy – but it also disguises many figure faults and will give you much needed confidence while you are awaiting the results of your diet and exercise programme.

Steps to a perfect posture

First try to stand correctly. Place your feet together or better still, as it is easier to balance, slightly apart and parallel, or with your heels together and feet forming a V-shape, at an angle of not more than 45 degrees, then:

- grip the floor or soles of your shoes with the pads of your toes and draw up your arches
- distribute your weight evenly between each foot, don't lean on one more than the other
- make sure the weight is spread slightly forward from the heels and concentrated across the instep and towards the outer borders and balls of your feet
- keep your knees straight but relaxed, not braced
- tuck your buttocks under, slightly squeezing the muscles
- tilt your pelvis so that the front part of the curved rim is directly above your pubic bone
- stretch your spine upwards, particularly the rib cage and neck, and expand your chest outwards slightly

- if the previous step is taken correctly, your shoulders should automatically fall into place, slightly further back and down
- your arms should hang loosely at your sides with the palms facing towards the back of outer thighs
- your ears should be level and directly above your shoulders and your shoulders should be level on each side
- tuck your chin in so that it is at right angles to your neck, your chin should neither be thrust forwards nor be tilted downwards
- the crown of your head should be the highest point of your whole body.

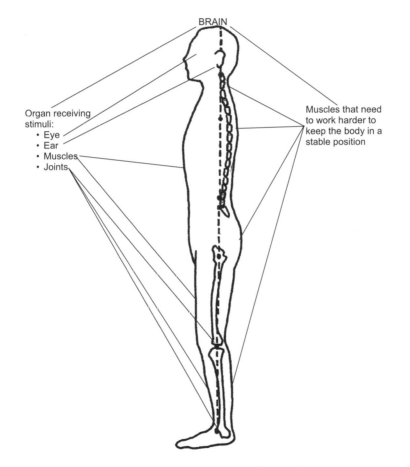

BRAIN

Organ receiving stimuli:
- Eye
- Ear
- Muscles
- Joints

Muscles that need to work harder to keep the body in a stable position

If you found any of the above difficult, it will reveal where your posture is incorrect. You will now need to practise corrective exercises to loosen any tight muscles and joints in the neck, chest, shoulders and lumbar spine.

Toning and strengthening weak muscles are good ways to begin postural improvement. You will find the neck side bends described below useful to release tension and increase the flexibility of your movements while alternate arm circling will help to correct round shoulders.

The pelvic roll, spinal curl and back slide will help to correct a too-deep hollow in the small of your back. This is often the cause of backache and discomfort around the abdomen and can become a contributory factor in digestive problems, constipation, varicose veins, hernia and prolapse of the womb. Don't be misled by the apparent simplicity of these exercises; they are among the most effective remedial exercises there are. The pelvic roll, in particular, is suitable for people of all ages and conditions, and is one of the first exercises given after an abdominal operation or as part of an antenatal or postnatal programme and forms the basis of more advanced abdominal exercises.

Incidentally this exercise was one of Elizabeth Arden's favourites which she demonstrated to me when as a slim lithe 80-year old she visited the London Salon where I was working at the time.

Neck side bends

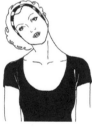

Bend your head and neck sideways, return to the centre then bend your head and neck to the opposite side. To correct any imbalance, repeat the exercise more frequently in the opposite direction to that of your usual tilt.

Alternate arm circling

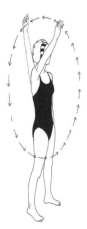

Alternately lift each arm forwards, up, backwards and down in a smooth circular motion. You can do this exercise from the standing or sitting position but keep the trunk erect and don't twist it from side to side.

Pelvic roll

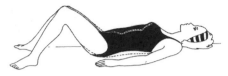

Lie on your back, with feet flat on the floor and knees bent to form a right angle. Tilt the lumbar spine against the carpet so that the top of the pelvis moves towards your trunk and the lower part of the buttocks rolls off the floor, while the pelvis remains in contact with it. At the same time draw your abdominal muscles inwards towards the spine to create a concave effect and press the shoulders down. Hold the contraction for 3 to 5 seconds, then relax. Breathe in to prepare, out as you contract, and in as you relax.

Spinal curl

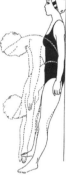

Stand with your buttocks against the edge of a wall or door jamb with heels a few inches forward from the edge of the floor, feet comfortably apart. Relax the trunk forward, bending gently at the knees. Now draw in the abdominal muscles and unwind the spine carefully, one vertebra at a time, without parting company with the wall or door. When you reach the chest area, be careful not to allow the lumbar vertebrae to lose contact (harder than it sounds). Drawing in the abdominal muscles more strongly will help.

Back slide

Stand with the back of your head and the entire back from the shoulders downwards against a wall or door. Your feet should be about 12 inches in front comfortably apart. Slide your spine down a few inches, then back up several times, bending and straightening the knees alternately (pointed over the feet), at the same time lifting and lowering the heels.

Posture in motion

As you become increasingly aware of your posture in daily life, you will be able to detect when you are holding your muscles too tightly (usually those in the neck, shoulders and lower back), and consciously 'let go'. It could be that you 'forget' to relax the muscles after carrying home shopping or tighten the muscles subconsciously when under stress. Once you have established the habit of using the muscles more economically, you will respond to stress or muscular activity with greater ease.

Even if you found it comparatively easy to stand correctly, practise at every available opportunity. Take a quick glance whenever you pass a mirror or shop window. Remember it is as easy to establish good habits as bad ones; it is just a question of repeating them often enough until they become automatic. Correct posture is not rigid. The only areas where muscles should be slightly tense are in the abdomen and buttocks. The rest of the muscles are stretched, especially above the waist and chest and again at the neck, but relaxed and fluid as long as the major joints are immediately above one another; for instance, ankles, knees, hips, shoulders and occipital joint where the head joins the neck.

Walking should be a continuation of this relaxed stance, flowing and easy with no awkward jerks. The weight should be drawn up through the legs to just above the waist to counteract the gravitational pull that causes the familiar heavy, dragging feeling. To experience the feeling of relaxed and balanced movement, practise the following exercises. Relax the knee of one leg, take a step by flexing the ankle and hip, then flex the foot and place first the heel and then the ball of the foot on the floor. The feet should be neither turned in nor turned out but point straight ahead. The space between each foot should be about half that of the width of the foot. Raise the heel of the other leg and repeat the movements. Your weight is being passed from heel to ball continuously, the emphasis being on the ball of the foot. As you complete each step, the knee is momentarily straightened and the hip is extended so that you should get a slight contraction in the buttock muscles.

Avoid unnecessary movement in the top of your body or in your arms. Try not to twist your trunk or sway from side to side, or lean to one side or the other. Don't let one shoulder rise higher than the other, which often happens when we carry things, or lean forward in a vain attempt to push yourself forward more quickly.

Improving everyday movements

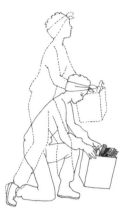

- When lifting anything heavy, bend your knees, not your back and put one knee on the floor near to the weight. Don't twist your trunk, but face the object squarely so that when lifting you distribute the weight of the object evenly. This also applies when carrying; always try to balance your shopping in each hand and don't allow the weight to pull you forward, or to one side. Try to keep your back, shoulders and head erect and hold the weight close to your body. Avoid resting a weight or child on one hip for any length of time.

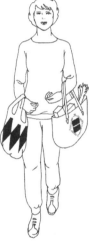

- When standing for long periods, you will find it less tiring if you relax the knees more than usual and place the feet further apart so that they are immediately under the hip joint. This will help avoid the tendency to lean on one leg or thrust the hips and pelvis forwards which accentuates the inward curve in the small of the back and pushes the abdomen forward, all of which will cause unnecessary strains. Supportive shoes with not too high a heel will also make it easier to stand comfortably, as will taking frequent small steps.

- Don't bend over working surfaces; they should be at a height that does not require too much bending over – ideally no lower than pelvis level. To raise the height, place say, a washing-up bowl on another upturned bowl, or on a draining board. To lower the height, place a suitable object on the floor to stand on. For other chores where you can sit, use a high stool.

- Kneel or squat for low jobs such as cleaning the bath or making beds. When sweeping or vacuum cleaning, don't twist your trunk violently from side to side or continuously bend the trunk forwards. Instead, face the broom or vacuum cleaner squarely.

- Always maintain an erect posture when using stairs, then it becomes an effective leg exercise, especially when going up. If necessary, use your nearest hand to hold the stair rail lightly for support. Place only the balls of the feet down as you take each step (not too near the edge). Keep the trunk, neck and head erect, tuck your buttocks under and draw your tummy well in. Avoid any tendency to lean forwards, sideways, or to place too much weight on the stair rail.

- When sitting, balance evenly on your buttock bones. Sit sufficiently back on the chair so that the small of your back is supported by the chair back, stretch your spine and neck upwards from the ribs, relax your shoulders and check that your jaw is at a right angle with your neck. Unless you are using your arms, they should be relaxed with hands resting on your lap. Your thighs should be fully supported by the chair seat and your trunk and thighs should form a right angle (at the hips) as should your thighs and lower legs (at the knees). Your feet should be placed flat on the floor, together for elegance, but hip width apart for comfort over long periods.

- Take care to avoid slumping or hollowing your back which will hinder your breathing and digestion. Don't cross your legs at the knees, particularly if you have circulatory problems such as varicose veins, as the pressure will delay the return of the blood to the heart. Avoid crossing your legs too if you suffer from a low back problem (lumbago or sciatica, for instance), because the hip and pelvic muscles will be used unevenly and thus aggravate your back. If the chair forces you to sit with an unnaturally curved lower back or round shoulders, simply sit further forwards. When working at a desk or table (reading or writing, for example), adjust your position, altering the desk or chair height if necessary, so that you don't raise one or other shoulder or grip the pen too tightly when you begin to tire. Prolonged sitting slows down the circulation, stiffens the hip and knee joints, cramps and shortens the muscles that flex the hips and knees, and also weakens and stretches the buttock and front of thigh muscles. If your work involves sitting, take a break now and again to move about and do some standing exercises.

- If your posture has been wrong for a long time, the correct posture is bound to feel strange and you will constantly have to make adjustments, especially when walking, sitting, standing at the sink or ironing-board, gardening, driving, sitting at a desk and so on. When new habits form, the adjustments will become increasingly instinctive. You may, however, have to check your posture when you are tired – this is when you are most likely to revert into a slump or to hollow your back.

- If you feel constantly tired or run down, it will be harder to hold yourself correctly. Assuming that you have your doctor's assurance that there is nothing medically wrong, perhaps you work too hard physically or mentally instead of trying to achieve a balance between the two. Perhaps you don't have sufficient recreation or relaxed sleep. Check your diet in case you lack some of the essential nutrients. Your neck, shoulder and back muscles may have tightened up through muscular or nervous tension. Treat your neck, shoulders and back to a massage or apply gentle heat from an infrared lamp or heat-pad and take a relaxing bath.

The correct way to breathe

Practise breathing easily and effortlessly. Breathing is largely an automatic function controlled by the brain, which receives and sends out messages so that the breathing rhythm is adapted, according to circumstances, to maintain the correct ratio of oxygen to carbon dioxide in the blood. If you force your lungs to expand unnaturally, and too quickly, you could feel tense, or slightly dizzy. Any sudden conscious alteration in the breathing pattern can upset the automatic mechanism and cause discomfort – you will avoid this if you take care to breathe more slowly than usual. Keep a relaxed feeling in the throat and allow the breath to deepen naturally. Pretend you are 'drinking' in the air and listen for a 'hissing' sound in the throat rather than a 'sniffing' sound in the nostrils. Aim to equalise the length of the in and out breath and allow the chest to expand easily and effortlessly.

With practice, your normal breathing rhythm will become slower and deeper and this will increase your sense of wellbeing. But keep a regular check throughout the day, especially when you are tense or tired. Breathing shallowly when tired or depressed, as most of us do, can increase these feelings; holding the breath or breathing unnecessarily fast when you feel uptight will also make you more tense.

Prolonged stress or the failure to channel stress into positive physical and mental activity, can also upset the natural rhythm of action, followed by a pause, as in the regular heart beat. This can affect any of the other automatic functions – circulation, endocrine glands, digestion and elimination. Many people think that because these systems operate mostly below conscious level, this means we have no control at all over them. But we can influence them indirectly by using the breath to help change a mood. This is possible because the nervous system and the endocrine glands that assist the brain to regulate the automatic functions are also involved with the emotions. When the mood changes, there is a response in the nerves and glands that affects all these functions and registers as a change in the breathing pattern.

Of all the body's vital systems, breathing is the one we have the most power to direct, so make full use of this power. Raise your level of awareness to any stress signals in the breath. Then, by breathing slowly and evenly you can help restore a sense of calm wellbeing, which will reflect as smoother functioning in the other systems.

Ill-effects caused by breathing badly include the following:
- If we are over-anxious, breathing becomes quick and we may tense and round the shoulders.
- This encourages shallow breathing as the lungs are not free to expand.
- If the back becomes 'fixed' in a humped position, this could cause depression from the less attractive appearance.
- Shallow breathing weakens the muscles that allow the lungs to ventilate fully, causing a vicious circle.
- As some of these muscles help to maintain an erect trunk and help to keep joints in the chest area flexible, this encourages a slumped posture still further.
- The bronchiole muscles can go into spasm, which makes breathing difficult and can manifest as asthma. The cause to some extent is nervous in origin, though it can be triggered by stimuli similar to those of hay fever, dust, pollen and feathers, for example.
- The mucous membranes, which line the respiratory tract, can become infected and clogged with excess mucus. This is interrelated with nervous tension and a diet lacking in foods rich in vitamins A and C, or containing too much sugar, starch and fats, or through smoking.

How you can correct the ill effects caused by breathing badly:

- Vigorous exercise, which creates an extra demand for oxygen, increases lung capacity as the muscles involved strengthen, and causes the opening up of more blood vessels in the lungs.
- Localised exercise to mobilise the shoulder girdle and strengthen the postural muscles that facilitate lung expansion by maintaining the body in an erect position.
- Consciously controlling the breath to exert either a calming or energising effect.
- Eating a nutritious diet rich in vitamins A and C (contained in yellow and orange fruits and vegetables, liver and fish-liver oils); controlling the intake of starches and fats; cutting out sugar and refined foods; and giving up smoking.

In addition to the use of breath to release tension here is a set of guidelines that I have found helpful to increase resistance to the harmful effects of too much stress.

Guidelines to increase resistance to the harmful effects of too much stress

The three basic essentials for health that can be applied to increase resistance to the harmful effects of too much stress are: (i) think right; (ii) eat right; (iii) move right.

- Recognise and accept the situation, whatever it is and distinguish between factors that can and cannot be changed. Accept yourself and others as you are and learn to work with, rather than against, circumstances.
- Constantly remind yourself that it is misuse that directs your vital energy to sickness and disharmony, and seek honestly to ascertain whether the situation could be due to a lack of knowledge or a negative attitude.
- Learn to work with other people, to anticipate and neutralise bad moods by side-stepping to avoid a head-on collision. Often there is tension, exhaustion or insecurity hidden under a bombastic or irritable surface.
- Keep a constant check on priorities and be willing to adjust them as circumstances change, and then concentrate on one thing at a time. This results in progress, satisfaction, and a willingness to relax.

79

- Try to divide the 24 hours into eight hours' sleep, eight hours' work, eight hours' recreation, then learn to recognise energy patterns, anticipate the onset of tiredness, and take a rest or change your activity. This helps prevent the inevitable swing of the pendulum from elation to tears or from extreme activity to exhaustion or boredom.
- Recognise the need to develop and balance the spiritual, mental and physical nature.
- Adopt a more realistic attitude to the use of time. Be flexible and don't necessarily fill every hour with a specific job or appointment. If time is set aside for thinking, browsing in a bookshop or visiting an art gallery, this time can be used where appropriate to meet an emergency.
- Analyse your motives if you are constantly trying to beat the clock; use your energy economically and don't use a 'sledge-hammer to crack a nut', nor use too much energy trying to impress others. If necessary, take longer to complete a task. Find a more efficient way of doing it, delegate or give up activities that no longer present a challenge. Watch your response to other people's demands. Consider carefully before making a commitment.
- Deal carefully with frustrations, neither suppressing them so that you become bitter, nor compensating unwisely. Work them out through a creative interest.
- Act confidently and follow up every good opportunity or any challenge that exhilarates you, even though you may feel a bit scared. Otherwise you will be plagued by regrets of what might have been, and may lose an exciting job or promotion.
- Learn to enjoy your own company. You are probably the most interesting person you know. So be gentle and give yourself the occasional treat. Then you will be able to be alone without being lonely. You will not be so reliant upon other people emotionally, and will be free to enjoy them more than ever before.
- Remember the power of thought. You need to attract the positive influences that will enable you to work through all your problems.
- Be aware of how climatic conditions affect you and take precautions to minimise discomfort.
- In cold weather, start the day warm. Wear thermal underwear if necessary.

Remember, several layers of clothing are better than one thick one. Cover the head and neck and, of course, hands so as not to lose unnecessary body heat. Wool is a good conductor of heat. Have a good protein breakfast with a little more fat than usual. Move more and quicker than usual. Close the pores with cool water after a hot bath or shower to keep body heat in.

- In hot and humid weather, wear loose cotton clothing. Move more slowly. Many people living in a temperate climate have sluggish sweat glands, so it is a good idea to stimulate gland activity now and then by a run, energetic work-out or a game, followed by a shower. Then make sure further perspiration evaporates as quickly as possible. This requires dry air or increased air velocity such as from a fan, from riding a bicycle, or from driving with the sun-roof open and wearing fewer, looser clothes made from cotton. Drink more liquids. Water-soluble vitamins and minerals (not just common salt) will be lost, so must be replaced. The loss of B vitamins in particular increases nervous and muscular tension, which produces more heat. At night, try an ice-cold water-bottle.
- Avoid unnecessary exposure to loud, strident noise by taking avoidance action where possible. Turn volume knobs down and muffle the telephone. Try wearing ear-plugs if you have to work near a busy street or in a noisy office.

Relaxation

Balancing the natural rhythms of effort followed by relaxation
Relaxation, according to the dictionary, means a diminution of tension or, to put it another way, a negation of effort. Relaxation can apply equally to the mind or body and does not necessarily imply sitting or lying down and doing nothing. It is possible to be actively engaged in work, in recreation or just sitting still in either a relaxed or tense manner.

The definition of tension is: being stretched, or mental strain or excitement. It can be good or bad, partly dependent upon the degree of tension.

Our ability to withstand stress varies a great deal. Stresses that some people would thrive on drive others to the point of nervous collapse. A healthy response to tension can increase physical and mental stamina and alertness and enables us to tap our creative resources, and increase confidence and the ability to solve problems. This peak condition can only remain if we leave sufficient time for relaxation and recreation, otherwise we could finally collapse from nervous and physical exhaustion.

Sooner or later we may respond negatively to these same tensions as harmful tension is the common denominator in all the killer diseases, if we value our lives, the priority must be to recognise it and take counteraction before the pattern is established and permanent damage done.

The rhythms of nature (heartbeat, respiration, night and day, and so on), suggest that our physical, mental and emotional energies should be used evenly and a period of activity followed by a period of rest. The secret is not to use one type of energy either for too long or too intensely and particularly not in a resentful or otherwise negative manner. Muscles are often held in a state of continuous contraction. The habit of relaxing, especially after repeated emotional response or the repeated lifting and carrying of heavy objects can easily be lost.

Excess tension is commonly found in the face, (eyes, temples, forehead, jaws), neck, shoulders, upper back, lumbar spine, hands and feet. It can be felt in various ways:
- Sensed in the form of headaches, neck, shoulder and backaches, and in irritability and increased fatigue.
- Felt as nodules or hardness in the muscles which tend to stand out.
- Seen in tense, rigid facial expressions and posture, and in awkward, jerky, perhaps exaggerated movements and emotional reactions, nail biting, finger tapping, irritability and impatience, for example.

Relaxation techniques can be used to increase both the recognition and release of nervous and muscular tension reflected in varying degrees of continuous contraction of particular muscle groups. This will lesson fatigue and have a revitalising effect, enabling energies to be used more positively and economically.

The following are examples which can be used to calm the nerves or increase vitality both during the course of daily life and during an exercise session. They will help rest tired muscles, enable the circulation to remove the chemical wastes from muscle work, and induce a sense of relaxation. Try out each method and then use them according to your own inclination and need. For the lying exercises, choose a carpeted floor with a flat cushion or rolled up towel under the pelvis, knees, head and neck, if necessary. If the floor is not carpeted, an exercise mat must be used.

Relaxation techniques
Soothing, relaxing music will help to set the mood and will be especially useful for the swinging and stretching movements. Breathe rhythmically and gently throughout.

Rhythmic swinging and pendular movements
Use gravity and momentum. Repeat each complete movement 6–10 times on one side and then on the other side.

Purpose: To encourage normal relaxation after effort (by incorporating reciprocal contraction of opposing muscle groups). Relieves habitual muscle tension and relieves mental tension by taking excess blood from the head.

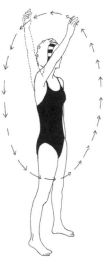

Shoulder circles
Stand or sit with arms relaxed by your side. Move the right shoulder forward, up, back and down in a circular movement. Repeat with the left shoulder.

Alternate arm circling
Stand or sit. Raise the right arm forward, up, back and down. Repeat with the left arm.

If the shoulder muscles are very tense, alternate arm circling may be too strong at first. If this is the case, swing one arm at a time forwards and backwards and side to side as with the leg swings below.

Forward and backward leg swings

Stand with the left hand resting lightly on a mantelpiece, shelf or similar support between shoulder and waist level. Swing the right leg forward and backward, straightening the knee gently on the forward swing and bending it gently on the backward swing. Turn around and repeat with the left leg.

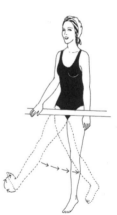

Side to side leg swings

Stand facing a support as in the previous exercise; rest both hands lightly on it. Raise the right leg forward a few inches, swing it to the right and then across in front of the left leg in a pendular motion. Repeat with the left leg.

Gentle stretches

Repeat each movement 3–4 times.

Purpose: To stretch tension gently out of the large muscle groups. Where you feel it most, indicates where the muscles are tense.

Shoulder pushes

Stand, sit, or lie on the back with feet flat and knees bent, and push both shoulders towards the feet for five seconds. Then stop pushing and allow the shoulders to recoil to their natural level. Notice if they are lower than before.

Gentle body stretch

Stand and raise the arms overhead. Reach up with the right arm while lifting the left heel, then with the left arm while lifting the right heel. This can also be done lying on the back with arms resting on the floor beyond the head. Push the right arm and left foot (with foot square to the leg) away from the trunk. Stop pushing and allow the muscles to recoil and relax. Repeat on the other side. If preferred, use the arm and leg on the same side.

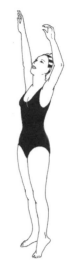

Scalp loosener

Using the pads of the fingers and thumbs of both hands, make small circular (shampooing-type) movements over the entire scalp.

Rhythmic breathing exercises

Sit comfortably on a chair, cross-legged or 'kneel sitting' on the floor. The throat should be consciously relaxed and air 'sucked' in with a gentle 'hissing' rather than 'sniffing' sound.

All breathing exercises unaccompanied by actual physical exercise should be performed more slowly than regular breathing and the length of the breath should be extended by slow degrees. This is to avoid upsetting the reflex mechanism which regulates the speed and depth of breath in order to maintain the correct ratio of oxygen to carbon dioxide in the blood. A sudden intake of oxygen can cause slight light-headedness and if the in-breath is forced, it could cause slight nervous tension.

Choose any or all of the following breathing exercises according to need:

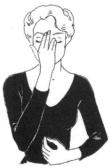

- Breathe slowly and effortlessly gradually allowing the breaths to become deeper and more vigorous – to increase vitality.
- As above, but close each nostril in turn, breathing out and in alternately with each nostril – will help

to balance active and sensing energies.
- Keep breathing especially gentle and effortless – to relax the nerves, steady the mind, and reduce the pulse rate.

After a few seconds, adjust the breath so that the in- and out-breaths are even in length. Continue practice for 5-10 minutes if possible.

Deep relaxation and meditation
Sit or lie in a comfortable position and continue to breathe gently and evenly:
- Try to visualise the body's innate healing energies easing areas of pain or discomfort.
- Try to recall and release emotional tension which may have been suppressed in the lower abdomen, solar plexus, chest, throat, forehead and temples.
- Concentrate on a word such as 'peace' either silently, or in the form of a chant (very effective in a group when, as vibrations become more in tune, the 'chord' becomes more harmonious).
- Concentrate on an object such as a cross, candle or flower, or mental imagery such as a country, sea or mountain scene.

It is difficult for some people to control their thoughts. The conscious mind will not actually stop working, but it is possible to guide it gently into a state of repose. It is even possible to raise the vibrations above conscious level into the realms of inspiration and vision.

Immediate and long-term effects of concentrated relaxation include:
- increased mental alertness and ability to concentrate;
- steadier mind and calmer emotions;
- lessening of aches and pains related to tension;
- increased energy and feeling of wellbeing;
- slower resting pulse and respiratory rates, lower blood pressure;
- gentler reactions to everyday situations and increased ability to cope with stressful situations without ill-effect.

Preparing for a good night's sleep

- Ideally, a period of recreation, however short, should follow the day's work, even if it is only switching on some soothing music or half an hour spent with an absorbing book.
- Start to unwind at least an hour before bedtime. Reflect briefly on the day's events, both good and bad, to get them into perspective. Acknowledge any problems demanding attention. Make notes and plans, particularly for the next day, and keep a pad and pen by the bed. Try to establish the order of priorities, but be prepared to change them where it appears necessary.
- Don't eat anything that you find indigestible near bedtime. If you do suffer from indigestion, the tissue salt Mag. Phos. will help relieve indigestion within minutes.
- Have a warm soothing drink without caffeine; try camomile tea, Instant Postum or dandelion coffee.
- Have a warm bath – avoid baths that are too hot, they can be over-stimulating.
- If you suffer from insomnia, instead of a conventional pill try one in homoeopathic form or take a herbal sleeping pill such as Passiflora. Calcium tablets with vitamin D and magnesium are also good; all these remedies are sold in herbalists or health food shops. Try a soft blue light or the tissue salts Combination B and Kali Phos. These remedies will help to restore a healthy nervous system, as will the B-complex vitamins and foods containing them.
- Sleep in a warm, well-ventilated, dark, quiet room if possible. If necessary, cut out the worst of street noise or other intrusive noise by using wax car-plugs.
- Your mattress should be firm, but not too hard, otherwise the small of the back cannot relax. Ironically it is on account of back trouble that most people are led into buying over-hard mattresses. Also avoid a lumpy bed with a dip in the middle.

Pillows are an individual matter. Unless you are actually suffering from chest trouble or an acute cold, when more may be necessary, one pillow is usually best. The back of the neck needs support, so sleeping without one could cause the neck to ache.

Many people choose to lie in a foetal position when preparing for sleep but this can easily cause discomfort in the neck, shoulders and lower back region.

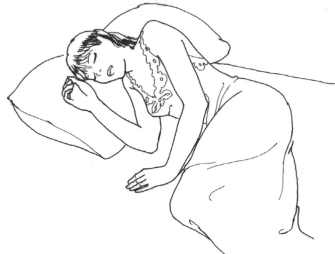

A better way to sleep if you choose to lie on your side is to bend the upper arm and knee and place the underneath arm and shoulder beside not under or in front of the trunk.

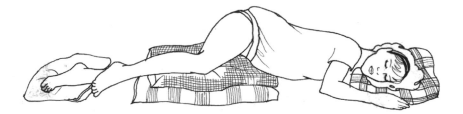

If you don't sleep the moment your head touches the pillow spend a few quiet moments breathing easily and gently. If sleep still seems to elude you, get up, walk about, read or write quietly. I may sit in my living-room and gaze at a painting with which I can identify and after a while I feel sufficiently tranquil to go to sleep.

A short night without tension is sufficient to get through the day in an efficient manner. I usually take an extra vitamin E tablet and another spoonful of honey at breakfast time the next morning to give my energy a boost, and the next night I drop off immediately my head touches the pillow.

Sleep is natural to the body, and the more we learn to relax – something that should be a continuous process through all the day – the deeper and more refreshing sleep becomes.

Individual needs vary. On average we need seven to eight hours a night, though many people manage on six during the week as long as they make it up at the weekends. Adults who need longer and would happily sleep at least nine to ten hours a night often suffer with low blood pressure or slight anaemia. Continuous insomnia, on the other hand, suggests there is something wrong with the way of life, either work or relationships. As we get older, on the whole we need less continuous sleep.

Remember that although the organs of the body (heart, lungs, digestive and eliminatory organs) are less active during sleep (a good reason for not eating a heavy meal late at night), the body chemistry continues to be very active, maintaining and repairing the cells. If we continually burn the candle at both ends, apart from tiredness, we shall age more quickly, simply because the cell renewal process will slow down. Be thankful for nature's pattern of day and night. Those of us who live life intensely must accept that nature intends us to live just one day at a time. Life is for living, not straining at the leash to prove we are indestructible. Sometimes more worthwhile things are achieved at a slower, more contemplative pace.

Constant tossing and turning is an indication of either physical or mental tension registering in the spine. Relax with some quiet floor exercises or in the yoga tranquil pose (below) before getting into bed.

Tranquil pose
Lie on the back, knees bent and soles of the feet resting on the floor and arms near sides. Breathe in, then while breathing out, roll the lumbar spine against the floor and lift hips and lower back off the floor. Pause to breathe in. While breathing out, tilt buttocks and legs towards the head. Legs will be

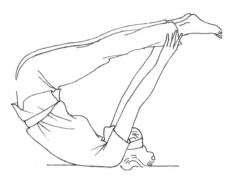

almost parallel to the floor and knees over the forehead. Raise the arms and place the hands on or below the knees, making any adjustments necessary to maintain balance. It may be more comfortable to relax the knees on to the forehead. Hold the position for at least three complete breaths and for two or three minutes, as long as you feel comfortable. Then, while breathing out, lower the legs to the floor, drawing the abdominal muscles in to prevent the spine and head from raising off the floor.

Yogis also suggest that we should arrange our bed so that we lie in line with the earth's magnetic flow from north to south and that this will have a balancing effect on the body. We should also lie on the side that enables us to breathe predominantly through the nostril that supplies either the active (right side) or receptive (left side) energies according to our specific needs, and change sides as these needs vary.

Everyday exercise and relaxation

Aware that my students had very little spare time, I introduced exercises that fitted into their daily activities. Why just do housework or dig the garden when you can exercise at the same time? Not only does being aware of how you hold and move your body during everyday activities mean that you build in exercise as an integral part of your life, but you will also gain more from the activity. And you are far less likely to end up with the aches and pains that follow strained movements. Some of these movements can also be adopted for use by office workers.

Housework

Get the full advantage from your housework! When making the bed, face it squarely without twisting the trunk. Protect your back by kneeling to tuck in the sheets and blankets instead of bending from the waist. Cleaning the bath may give your back a twinge. Kneel, if you can, and draw your abdominal muscles well in so that they take part of the strain. Afterwards when you straighten up, take a good stretch. Better still, try cleaning the bath before getting out.

Welcome dusting and polishing jobs, especially those where you have to reach up. Use your arms as vigorously as you can and swap hands from time to time to give yourself the opportunity to firm the arms and chest muscles on both sides of the body. The same benefits can be gained from washing or polishing a floor by hand. Each time you wash up do some press-ups against the sink unit. Bend the knees, not the back, when opening low drawers and cupboards. Every time you sweep a floor use the broom handle to do trunk twists, side bends and shoulder straighteners. When using a vacuum cleaner or floor sweeper be careful to face it straight; it is very easy to give the back a twinge by uncontrolled swinging and twisting movements. When passing a full length mirror, check your posture and lift from the ribs, tuck your buttocks under and draw the abdominal muscles in.

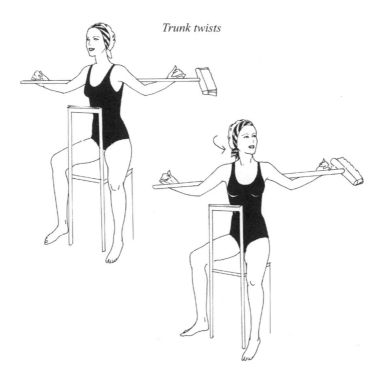

Trunk twists

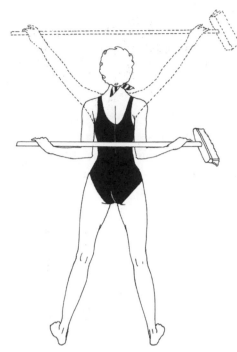

Shoulder straightener

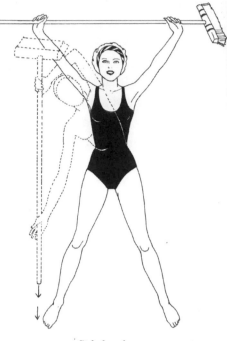

Side bends

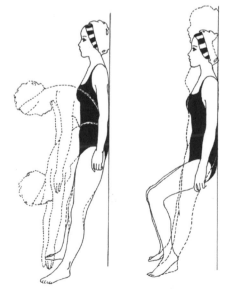

Spinal curl   *Back slide*

At least twice a day, unwind your spine against the corner of a door frame or cabinet to correct the tendency to a hollow back which nearly all of us have. You can also press the entire back flat against the smooth surface of a door frame, wall, or filing cabinet and slide up and down several times. Then, with the calves at a right angle to the thighs, hold the position, pull your abdominal muscles well in and press your lumbar spine into the surface; as well as relaxing your spine, this will also strengthen your thigh muscles. When waiting for your tea or coffee to cool, do some breathing exercises.

In the bath

An opportunity to do your neck exercises and ankle circles. You could use one hand to circle your toes in each direction and give a gentle pull, then spread the toes wide apart and if you are tall enough, press the sole of the foot against the end of the bath and draw up the arches. Exercise the calf muscles by pressing the ball of the foot against the end of the bath and raising the heel up. For the abdomen, place the soles of the feet firmly on the bottom of the bath and do a few bent knee sit-ups. Then, as you pull out the plug, stand up without using the arms, if possible. Alternatively, get up using your arms if you think they also need firming.

Gardening

As with cleaning out cupboards and drawers indoors, if you insist on doing one job over a prolonged period, it can become back-breaking. It is always best to switch jobs and positions at regular intervals; then have a good stretch before continuing. So with gardening, when weeding you can alternate between squatting and kneeling (on a comfortable mat). Try not to bend forward; twisting is all right as long as the back is straight. Digging is marvellous for arms and legs but keep the trunk as straight as possible.

Hoeing seems easy by comparison but be careful of uncontrolled twisting if you suffer with low backache. Try to face the hoe straight on or you may ache for days. If you are planning to cut the hedge, first do some alternate arm circling to make sure your shoulders are flexible. Using shears will firm the arm and chest muscles. Do not carry on for too long without a pause to stretch and relax the arms.

In the swimming pool or sea

Working against the resistance of the water will increase the effectiveness of some of the exercises. Working with the buoyancy of the water will of course take the strain from the joints and make some movements easier. Start with 5 repetitions and gradually increase them according to need and ability.

To firm the outer thighs and hips lie on your side and grasp the rail, press the underneath leg down as far as possible.

To firm the inner thigh, same position but push the top leg down.

To firm front of thigh and lower abdomen grasp the rail and lie on your front; either bend the knees alternately to the chest or lift alternate legs with the knees straight, always be sure to round the back and carefully draw the abdominal muscles in.

To firm the buttocks, grasp the rail and lie on your back, alternately press each leg downwards.

To firm the front of the thighs stand in the shallow end of the pool and grasp the rail, alternately bend each knee and lift the leg, then straighten the knee with the ankle flexed (i.e. the foot square to the leg).

To firm the waist grasp the rail and lie on the back, move both legs first to one side then to the other, so that there is a side movement in the spine; from the same starting position, rotate the pelvis as far as possible from side to side.

On the beach or in the garden with friends or family

Games one and two are suitable for team games. Games two and three are more suitable for those who can do sit-ups easily. These are only a few suggestions there are endless possibilities and you may be inspired to make up your own.

1. Line up in two teams (you will need two balls for this game) so that a ball can be passed alternately overhead and between the legs, and each person is able to get a good stretch and bend (increases trunk flexibility). The last person runs with the ball to the front. Repeat until the first person is in front again. The first team to finish wins.
2. Another team game, only suitable for dry weather. The teams lie on their backs toes to head. Each person raises their arms to a right angle with the trunk. The ball is passed by sitting up and bending forward to place it in the hands of the person in front, then unwinding the spine carefully back to the ground (firms abdominal muscles). An easier alternative is to remain sitting so that when the last person receives the ball, he or she

bends forward, sits up again, slowly unwinds to the ground and passes it into the hands of the person sitting behind, and so on.

3. Another version of the above. Everyone lies down in a large circle with their feet towards the middle. The person with the ball calls a name, both people sit up and the ball is thrown and caught (hopefully), then they unwind to the ground (firms the abdominal muscles). The person with the ball then calls out another name and so on.

4.

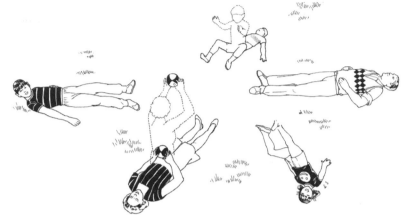

The 'hip walk' is great fun used as a race. Everyone sits on their buttocks, with legs straight and together, then 'walks' forward on each buttock in turn, lifting each leg entirely off the ground (knees straight and feet at a right angle with the legs if possible), over a pre-planned course; continue the race backwards to the starting point (firms muscles in the lower abdomen, waist and front of legs – if knees are kept straight; stimulates circulation through friction on buttocks).

The above exercises can be adapted for just two people and will work best if they are of similar heights.

In the classes we also had great fun trying out the following masks and the face exercises that follow.

Masks for all skin types

If you have a normal to dry skin, for best results you need to use a face mask every two weeks, once a month at the outside. If you have a spotty or oily skin, use a mask once or twice a week. For a combination skin, apply the mask only to the spots or oily patches. It is not advisable to apply a mask on the day of, or the day before, any special occasion unless spots are already dry, because it will draw them to a head so that temporarily they will be more noticeable. Always cleanse and tone the skin prior to using a mask, and if you have a dry skin and the mask itself contains no oil, first massage in a little of your normal night cream. A good mask will cleanse deeply by stimulating circulation and bring impurities to the surface; it will also feed the skin in varying degrees according to the type of ingredients used.

Dry skin

Mix one egg yolk with approximately one tsp of oil (almond or other vegetable oil) and add a little yeast powder (optional). Smooth on to the skin with a wooden spatula or a spoon or fork handle; take it well round the neck and down to the 'V' line of the chest but avoid the area around the eyes. Leave it on for 15–20 minutes (preferably lie down and rest during this time), then remove as much as possible with the spatula. Gently sponge away the residue with lukewarm water. Recleanse the face and splash with water or spray on spring water or tonic. Tissue dry and apply moisturising cream. Try not to use make-up for the rest of the day or for at least several hours after using a mask.

Dry or normal skin

Mix one egg yolk, 2 dessertspoonsful/40 ml of top of the milk or cream, one dessertspoonful of dried skimmed milk powder. Apply and remove in the same manner as above.

Sensitive skin

Mix one tbsp wheat germ with one tbsp plain yogurt.

Oily skin

Whisk one egg white and combine with sufficient fine oatmeal to make a paste.

For bleaching the skin if very sallow

Mix one tbsp lemon juice, one tbsp 20 vol. peroxide and one tsp glycerine.

As an alternative, simply massage in buttermilk or plain yogurt and leave on overnight, if possible.

For firming and moisturising
Mix one egg white, one tsp orange juice and one tsp honey.

Moisturising
Mix one dessertspoon almond or other vegetable oil, one dessertspoon honey and approximately half an average-length cucumber, grated. Place a tissue or gauze over this mask once in place to stop it running.

Honey acne lotion
Dissolve one dessertspoon honey in ½ pt./284 ml warm water, add 2 tsp lemon juice or cider vinegar. Bathe the affected skin with this mixture night and morning. The lotion will also help to soften boils and heal wounds.

Quick relievers

Burns or grazes	– apply honey.
Bags under the eyes	– half a slice of cucumber placed under the eyes.
Sunburn or freckles	– apply plain yogurt or buttermilk.
Spots (i)	– apply Boracic powder, which will help to dry them.
Spots (ii)	– apply Marmite or other yeast extract and cover with a waterproof plaster (the simplest remedy of all).

Face exercises
Laughing and chewing are by far the best exercises for the face muscles. Exercises that entail frowning and other exaggerated movements all too often encourage unnecessary lines, and although there is a wide selection of possible facial exercises, they are best done under close supervision. Here are one or two safe ones. Do them when comfortably seated.

Open wide

Purpose:	To tone muscles in the cheeks and around the eyes and jaw.
Method:	Open mouth and eyes as wide as possible; relax.

Repetitions: 5

Progressions: • Increase repetitions to 10 or more.

• Hold wide open position for 3 seconds, later increasing to 5 seconds.

Cheek blow

Purpose: To tone the cheek muscles.

Method: With a closed mouth, blow out the cheeks then suck them in.

Repetitions: 5

Progressions: Increase repetitions to 10 or more.

OOh-ick

Purpose: To tone the cheek muscles.

Method: Say or mouth 'ooh-ick' as forcefully as possible.

Repetitions: 5

Progressions: • Increase repetitions to 10 or more.

• Hold the 'ooh', then the 'ick' for 3 seconds, increasing later to 5 seconds.

Jaw moving 1

Purpose: To tone muscles around the mouth and jaw.

Method: Purse lips and move the jaw alternately to the right and left.

Repetitions: 5

Progressions: Hold to the right, then to the left for 3 seconds, later increasing to 5 seconds.

Jaw moving 2

Purpose: To tighten the lower jaw and throat muscles.

Method: With a closed mouth, lower the bottom jaw as far as possible.

Repetitions: 5

Progressions: • Increase repetitions to 10 or more.

• After lowering the jaw as far as possible, hold for 3 seconds, later on for 5 seconds.

Smile

Purpose: Similar to 'Open wide' exercise.

Method: Sit with the elbows resting on a table surface, heels of the hands just beyond the outer corners of the eyes, fingers pointing upwards. Push the skin of the cheeks up slightly with the heels of the hands, open the mouth and eyes wide, then close them.

Repetitions: 5

Progressions: • Increase repetitions to 10 or more.

                  • Hold 'wide open' position for 3 seconds, later increasing to 5 seconds.

The following 'exercises' cover several important meridian points used in aromatherapy and have a wonderful detensing effect; they are useful in helping to relieve or cure a headache.

Using either the middle or ring fingers, make gentle circling movements for a second or two on each of the following points, then repeat the routine several times.

1 Outside corners of the eyes (further in than the temples).
2 Under the centre of the eyebrow arch.
3 Inner corners of the eyes.
4 The 'knobs' on either side of the nose.
5 The outside of the nostrils.
6 Under the centre of the cheek-bones.
7 Vertically down from the above point, level with the corners of the mouth.
8 Midway between the nostrils and the centre of the upper lip.

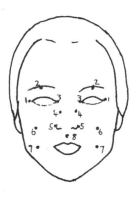

chapter 11

My search for a personal philosophy

Icontinued teaching these courses for several years until my job in a health club involved evening work. I was still at the health club in March 1963 when my father died unexpectedly and shortly afterwards I had an experience that reaffirmed my belief in life after death. I was on a bus and met a lady with whom I'd worked while at the Red Cross. She had just lost her sister and gave me copies of booklets written by Lady Dowding, the widow of Air Chief Marshall Sir Hugh Dowding who led the RAF to victory in the Battle of Britain in 1940. During his lifetime, they often communicated telepathically and had decided that whoever died first would try to communicate telepathically with the one left behind to describe life after death. While reading the booklet, I immediately felt uplifted into another dimension, the same feeling I'd had when after my father's death I 'knew' he was very close to me. The words had the ring of truth as if I was getting confirmation of what I already 'knew'. Briefly, the little booklet suggested that when we 'die' loved ones draw near to help us through the transition, after which we review the life just lived and then gravitate to souls on a similar wave length and continue to learn and serve in spirit unfettered by a physical body. At the time I tried to discuss these ideas with the local vicar and later with other clergymen especially when I came to believe in reincarnation, but I hit a brick wall because these ideas did not fit with their dogma.

My own search for a living philosophy took me beyond the confines of a particular creed. Although I was fortunate to grow up in an environment based firmly on Christian principles, I felt the need to go beyond the dogma of organised religion to find satisfying answers to some of life's more puzzling questions. The broad precepts that I have come to live by help me as much to sort out my priorities in daily life and to make positive decisions as they do to cope with more serious crises. Everyone must find their own beliefs, but I am sharing mine with you because if you read them with an open mind, you will respond more positively to the practical advice offered. Even if you disagree violently with some of my ideas, at least you may be stimulated to form a clearer picture of your own beliefs.

> *Our birth is both a sleep and a forgetting,*
> *The Soul that rises with us our life's Star,*
> *Hath had elsewhere its setting,*
> *And cometh from afar;*
> *Not in entire forgetfulness,*
> *And not in utter nakedness,*
> *But trailing clouds of glory do we come*
> *From God, Who is our home.*
> William Wordsworth, *Ode on Imitations of Immortality.*

The possibility of reincarnation

The realisation that we cannot work through the effects of all our mistakes, let alone become 'perfect' in one life, finally led me to a belief in reincarnation. It is an essential part of some world religions but as yet not part of the Christian doctrine, although references in the Bible suggest that Christ, Himself, accepted it. When speaking of John the Baptist, he implied several times that John was a reincarnation of Elijah:

> *And if ye will receive it, this is Elias, which was for to come.*
> Matthew, *Chapter 11, Verse 14.*

> *But I say unto you, that Elias is come already, and they knew him not, but have done unto him whatsoever they listed. Likewise shall also the son of man suffer of them.*
> Matthew, *Chapter 17, Verse 12.*

The idea of reincarnation is difficult to prove but we often hear of incidents which suggest it to be true. A well known example is that of the authoress, Joan Grant, who wrote books on Ancient Egypt that were amazingly accurate about matters she had not studied and which were afterwards verified by scholars. She actually claimed that in an earlier incarnation she had been an Egyptian princess and it would be difficult to explain the facts by any other theory.

I believe there are many dimensions or planes of experience in the unseen world (just as there are on the earth plane) though at a higher vibrational level. They may even occupy the same space as the visible universe and all interpenetrate with one another. We have all experienced telepathy, perhaps unknowingly, to some degree and as we develop our higher intuitional centres, we become increasingly sensitive to these unseen influences.

In sleep, I believe our spirit 'body' (soul) is able to leave the physical body and travel to higher planes to receive guidance and meet other souls, both those still on earth and those who are not, although we may be unaware of this in our conscious mind. Just as on earth we gravitate to people on a similar wavelength, so do we in the unseen world both during sleep and when we 'die'. Whereas on earth we can hide behind a veneer, in the spirit world I believe our thoughts will be transparent and more powerful so that we shall be able to project ourselves to different places by thought alone.

As we progress spiritually, we shall be able to reach higher planes and eventually no longer need to return to an earth life. Perhaps we may even learn the mysteries of creation and participate in them.

I believe that in any one life we incarnate only a part of our real self. Most of our higher mind and spirit remains in the higher dimension. But we can draw on its wisdom from beyond conscious level through prayer, meditation and during sleep. It is through this higher mind which, I believe, is linked to the Universal Mind (God) that we are sometimes able to recognise instantaneously the truth of new ideas without need of logic, as if remembering something we already know.

Group souls
Some people may wonder why an earth life is necessary at all. It is probably the very restrictions of earth which provide the widest possible experience

to learn our toughest character lessons, a process requiring many lifetimes. I believe that souls are created in groups, individual souls being bound to each other in order to fulfil a specific group destiny taking, perhaps, many thousands of lifetimes. If we remain spiritually asleep or continually fail to use opportunities for soul-development, we become 'lost' and sick. This can cause us to lag behind, or even delay the progress of the group, until we are spiritually awakened and restored in body and soul to continue our earth training and purpose. I believe we return as members of different races and religions, sometimes as a male, sometimes as a female, in similar groups but in differing relationships with each other so that our mother in one incarnation might be our brother in another, for example.

After death and preparation for rebirth

When we 'die', I believe loved ones in the other dimension draw close to help us through the transition. We then review the life we have just lived and rest awhile before continuing to learn and serve in spirit unfettered by a physical body. Present day hypnotists, practising regression therapy, have demonstrated that some of the deep memories revealed by patients under hypnosis appear to be those of previous lives. Evidence suggests that although it is possible for a soul to be reborn within a few years of death, the period between lives is more likely to be several hundreds of years in earth time.

The time for our return to another earth life is predetermined (according to the purpose for which we were created) so that we re-enter at the right point in history. As a preparation, we gather certain of our talents and mental resources attained in a previous life to help us in our task; our parents, racial background, other souls in our group are all selected and we are given a picture of the main lessons and situations to be encountered. While on earth, this blueprint is stored in the recesses of the mind and most of us only get glimpses of it as we plan our future and reach major turning points in our lives. Our happiest and most contented moments are probably those that give us a subconscious glimmer that we are fulfilling our destiny. This is even more true of those who pursue a vocation with an energy and dedication that leaves others gasping; perhaps they know that there is no other way to find peace of mind. Such beliefs also help to explain the immediate rapport we can experience with someone on a first meeting, feelings of having 'been there before', being more at home in some countries or districts than others, having a 'feel' for specific periods of history and so on.

The bread we cast upon the waters, good and bad, will eventually return, although the process is not always completed in one lifespan. This may be the reason that we sometimes face problems that we do not seem to have precipitated in this life. Karma is the term used in Eastern philosophy to refer to the sum total of causes set in motion in past lives as well as the current one, determining present conditions and providing opportunities for us to change for the better. Thus, if we harm others intentionally, we have to learn our mistake from a similar experience, though if, through ignorance or misunderstanding, harm befell another, the repercussions would not be so great. Equally, by acting with goodwill, we will eventually receive similar goodwill. Destiny is our potential, the plan which is in our power to fulfil. Fate is the degree of fulfilment not just the effects of past causes, but what we make of them. It is not necessarily inevitable, as it is always in our power to modify the effects of our reactions. Whether we allow ourselves to be crushed or use our opportunities for good is entirely up to us. Although we are predestined to work out our problems in the condition in which we find ourselves, we can use free will to determine future causes and thus shape our future destiny.

Everyone must find their own guidance: for me it is a God who is both good and in ultimate control, although I also accept that we are unlikely to find all the answers to our queries in this life. Even so, I think there is sufficient evidence of a higher intelligence and of laws operating within the apparent chaos to suggest that tragedy and disaster may sometimes be the culminating effects of the past. God gives us a certain amount of free will to evolve consciously through experience, and he is too immense to be interpreted in human terms, bargained with or placated.

The source of life
I believe in an Infinite Source and that can be interpreted in many ways and by different convictions. If there are individual forms of life, individual

forms of energy, different individual expressions of energy, there must be a source from which they come. I believe this energy flows in an orderly manner and according to set laws or patterns. One law to understand is Cause and Effect, which we can see embodied in many proverbs: we reap what we sow. If we can use the experience, then we will be all the better, yet even such a simple law can have its mystery.

Spiritual laws

Space does not allow for an in-depth explanation of such spiritual laws but here follows a list of some of the most significant ones:

Law of love	Which binds together matter and spirit from the atomic level upwards, everything in creation working in harmony.
Law of light	Which illuminates our minds and souls so that we can recognise spiritual truths.
Law of harmony	Which establishes balance by means of the mutual attraction of opposites (as with the positive and negative poles in electricity).
Law of attraction	By which like attracts like to establish a degree of order and enables us to draw opportunities to fulfil our needs.
Law of cause and effect	Whereby we reap what we sow.
Law of karma	Whereby we meet obstacles and situations, many pre-ordained, being the result of our actions in previous lives that present us with opportunities to change for the better.
Law of evolution	Whereby each level of creation makes its own contribution helped by the level above (spiritual, human, animal, plant, mineral) and slowly develops an awareness of the mysteries of creation.

The Source (God) is absolute, perfect and self-contained. Everything else is created from it and relative to it. I think of Creation as the pouring out of God's spirit to create in his own image (Oneness, the Infinite Source that continuously manifests itself as divisions of itself) and evolution as a going out and a coming back (a continuous process until every part recognises its true origins, consciously seeks and eventually reunites with them).

We have within our soul ('spirit body') a fraction of the Infinite Source, our Real Self or Spirit which is absolute and lives forever, one day to be reunited with the Source. Everything else in our body and mind, in fact everything in creation, is relative to the absolute and originates from the same source. So we are linked from within ourselves to that source, and we can draw upon these resources in order to overcome all our difficulties.

When we lose our sense of being in touch with the Source, we succumb to negative feelings and become unable to cope. It is not that we are not linked to God, simply that we **think** we are not, so cannot use the help that is there all the time.

Ten steps to a personal philosophy

1. We are all created from the same source, God, the Infinite Source. If there are individual forms of life, individual forms of energy, there must be a source from which they come. This concept helps us to recognise the Oneness of Nature and to respect all parts of the whole: the elements, rocks, minerals, plants, insects, fishes, animals, humans as well as the spiritual unseen world.

2. We are inherently linked to the Source within our own soul but we must keep the communication lines open with such activities as prayer, meditation, the enjoyment of uplifting music, literature and art and taking part in ventures for the good of the community. We can feel separated from the Source when we use our physical, emotional, psychic, mental and spiritual energies unevenly or negatively, either too much, too little or destructively.

3. Creation is a continuous happening, energies pouring forth ceaselessly; new stars and life systems being born on the edge of the Universe; the Infinite Source continually manifesting as divisions of itself on many planes and dimensions of existence other than the visible world, on differing wavelengths and vibratory frequencies. Resources are

limitless; mankind's problem is in learning how to use them wisely and in a balanced way.

4. Evolution is the continuous going out and coming back until each part of creation recognises its origins and consciously seeks to reunite with it, each level being helped by the one above to reach a state of awareness of its origins and purpose. More evolved beings in the spiritual world help us to make our contribution to life, and we in turn should help the animal kingdom and other forms of life on earth to do the same. As we evolve, our concept of truth will deepen and expand, inevitably leading to changes within our being and outer circumstances.

5. Light (energy in movement) is life – sunlight, mental light, spiritual light. The energies given forth by the sun produce vibrations that are converted into light waves as they penetrate the earth's atmosphere. Everything on the planet is made of and also emits these vibrations (electro-magnetic energies). On a mental level we talk of 'throwing light' on a subject. In the Bible Christ was described as the 'Light of the World'. The Universe is an ocean of movement, the motion of the earth and planets creates the gravitational force that keeps them in space. If the movements stopped the planets would collapse. Lack of movement, stagnation in any area is eventual death. On a physical level, cell renewal slows down, organs degenerate, muscles atrophy, joints stiffen. When the heart stops and we stop breathing, we die. Thus, if we don't move progressively on a mental and spiritual as well as physical level, our life slowly degenerates – maybe fate tries to shock us into positive action before it is too late.

6. We are what we think, that is, we are the sum total of what we believe. We can only use, enjoy and co-operate with the forces we recognise: truths, energy patterns such as the orderliness of planetary movements, astrological influences, biorhythms, natural laws such as gravity, spiritual laws such as cause and effect –- we reap what we sow. So beware of a closed mind. Albert Einstein believed that all matter is thought vibrating at a lower frequency, so perhaps it is not too far-fetched to suggest that God had an inspired thought and poured forth His Spirit in the form of energies which by transmutation into all the many elements became the Universe.

107

7. Thought patterns like movement patterns are registered in the brain. If a previous incident was misunderstood, so will each similar subsequent one be. Watch for these possibilities and try to correct them by asking the subconscious mind (where all our past memories and habits are stored) to send them up for review.

8. We must accept responsibility for the consequences of our thoughts and actions (the effects of all our causes) and, when things go wrong, not place all the blame on circumstances or other people; be aware of the fallibility of human beings, including our own. Apart from national disasters over which we have much less control on a personal level, we should examine each situation as objectively as possible to determine whether a negative attitude or gap in our knowledge contributed to the problem, and then aim to correct our errors.

9. There is always a lesson to be learned. Until it is, history repeats itself and a chain reaction is set in from past events finally culminating in the present event. We must also learn to combat influences under which negative emotions such as fear, hate and greed delay our progress.

10. Each soul on entering the earth plane has subconscious access to characteristics, skills and mental capabilities accumulated in previous lives. Since I cannot accept that we can work through the effects of all our causes or become 'perfect' in one life, I believe we return to an earth life many times. Reincarnation is an essential part of some world religions, but not yet part of the Christian doctrine, although references in the Bible suggest that Christ Himself accepted it.

Thirteen guidelines for problem solving

When a problem arises, here is a set of guidelines that I have found effective:

1. Try to pause, an immediate sigh or out breath will act as a brake, then take in and accept what has actually happened, distinguishing between what can and cannot be changed. Then consciously breathe slowly, gently and evenly to calm the nerves. This helps restore the feeling of unity with the Universal Mind and will disperse any negative emotion, making it impossible to feel resentment or apprehension, for example.

2. Avoid over-reacting. Speaking or acting too soon can be more disastrous than the event. Our reactions may, to some extent, be influenced by such things as the weather, our menstrual cycle or biorhythms, or the phases of the moon, but most of all by how uptight or tired we are.

3. Lessen tension by a positive thought – a smile instead of a frown. If a friend has let you down, immediately tell yourself there is probably a good reason that will eventually come to light. Learn to direct your thoughts rather than be controlled by them.

4. If the problem is a cancelled date, appointment or holiday, try to fill in the time you have unexpectedly been given as profitably as possible – there is always a silver lining.

5. If the answer to the problem is not immediately obvious, say a prayer. A prayer is a spiritual thought and to be effective, it should be a calm but concentrated request for help. It is the sincerity and depth of concentration that is important – not the length. Keep an open mind; don't presume to know what the answer **should** be, only desire to know the 'right' solution.

6. If the problem disturbs you, read from your own personal collection of 'truths' or from the Bible or other spiritual text.

7. If you have a favourite technique such as meditation, put it into practice. Relax and concentrate for 10–20 minutes on a suitable word or phrase to steady the conscious mind. For example: I am a part of the Universal Mind and can attract like a magnet all the help I need. This will link you to your higher mind (the superconscious), which in turn is linked with the Universal Mind-Source and open the way for intuitive thoughts to be received. Don't be disappointed if they don't come immediately.

8. Sometimes all that is required is a walk in a quiet atmosphere, to listen to some uplifting or soothing music, or to have a long sleep.

9. As soon as possible, examine the facts. Beware of misjudging the situation as a result of hurt pride or nervous tiredness. What we think are facts can be wrong opinions.

10. Look for contributory causes: these are usually interrelated and may include exhaustion, lack of knowledge and negative attitudes where fear is usually at the root.

11. Sometimes it helps to talk to a friend, but remember that the help of a

reputable therapist or counsellor can offer a wise and more unbiased view when dealing with a serious problem.

12. Accept the responsibility for what has happened. Face the worst that can happen. Then accept the lesson to be learned once it is found.
13. List all possible solutions (pros and cons). Now delegate all these details for the attention of the subconscious mind. At the same time, open up to the higher superconscious in order that a solution can be worked out. This procedure involves great control. Tensing-up must be avoided otherwise you will be unable to 'hear' the answer when it comes.

If the previous steps have been followed, eventually the solution (short or long term) will emerge with the assistance of your super- and subconscious minds. Should the solution take longer than expected, retrace your steps, then do the next thing that seems right. If still uncertain, wait until an opportunity or a growing intuition to present themselves. The time may not yet be ripe, but be ready to act when it is. We often have to wait patiently for the right circumstances. This is where trust in the unseen for our ultimate good is absolutely necessary.

For the future, learn to anticipate vulnerable situations and take any necessary steps to avoid recurrence of the same problem.

> *Truth is within ourselves; it takes no rise*
> *From outward things, whate'er you may believe.*
> *There is an inmost centre in us all,*
> *Where truth abides in fulness; and around,*
> *Wall upon wall, the gross flesh hems it in,*
> *This perfect, clear perception – which is truth.*
> *A baffling and perverting carnal mesh*
> *Binds it, and makes all error: and to KNOW*
> *Rather consists in opening out a way*
> *Whence the imprisoned splendour may escape,*
> *Than in effecting entry for a light*
> *Supposed to be without.*
>
> Robert Browning, *Paracelsus.*

Happy days at Elizabeth Arden
and ending the co-dependent relationship

Two months after my father's death, a girl at the health club took a job as a make-up artist at the Elizabeth Arden Salon in Bond Street and told me there was a vacancy for an exercise teacher. She suggested I applied for it, which I did and was immediately offered the job. It began in May 1963 and revealed my ability to communicate and demonstrate to a wide selection of the community. Having had an initial training in exercise therapy from the resident physiotherapist at the health club, I slipped into the work with ease and was taken aback when I was congratulated for explaining to clients the precise purpose of the specific exercise chosen for them. To me this was elementary. How could I expect clients to have faith in me or the exercise if they didn't understand what the exercises were intended to achieve! All the well-known film stars, pop stars and actresses of the period came to the salon. I remember teaching Cilla Black leg exercises, massaging Lee Radziwill (Jacqueline Kennedy's sister) and teaching yoga to Ava Gardiner to name but a few. Shirley Bassey, Elaine Stritch, Una Stubbs and Gayle Hunnicutt regularly visited our department as did Princess Margaret. When she had her children, the masseuse who treated her at Kensington Palace asked me to supply suitable post-natal exercises which I did. One day when I was being overworked, no lunch, tea or coffee breaks, I shut my door in desperation and escaped to the canteen for a quick snack. Trust my luck that during this time, H.R.H., as she was known, emerged from her treatment with the manageress and enquired 'What is behind that door?' The manageress having complete faith in me, opened my door and was faced with absolute chaos, records strewn on the floor, clients' record cards likewise and maybe even a record playing. H.R.H. apparently exclaimed 'Oh dear, what a mess!' Needless to say the manageress was overcome with embarrassment and afterwards sent for me to explain myself. Happily, this was the only time I put a foot wrong in my time at the Salon.

Between 1967 and 1970 Jack, the artist made a brief return into my life. Throughout the years we've always come together when one or both of us were in need, as if our souls were calling out to each other. He called me at Elizabeth Arden's out of the blue having met an uncle of mine by chance in Bond Street and asked where I was. His marriage had been difficult from the outset and my relationship with Dennis was reaching crisis point. We were able to meet occasionally and correspond during this period and one day he asked me whether I thought we should have married. To me the answer was an obvious yes, but I dared not say so for fear of bursting into tears, which I know would have happened. At the same time I was thinking if he truly loved me he wouldn't need to ask such a question. In any event, I bottled it and replied weakly that I didn't know.

Further examples of help from an invisible source

During this difficult period, I had two experiences which alerted me to the availability of other forms of help. The first example involved an urgent phone call I needed to make to a client. Outgoing calls had to be made through the main operator, but in this instance I was kept waiting and the operator never answered me. After a while I heard a click down the phone, then the ringing tone and to my amazement, the person who answered was the client I was trying to reach. This occurred without any human involvement. Was this the result of my own positive thought, or possibly the intervention from the spirit world? In the other example I had been sent by the salon to massage a lady who lived in the heart of Hampstead Heath. Taxis were arranged to take me and return me to Bond Street for my next client, but the return taxi never arrived. I was stranded in a very lonely part of the Heath, with no available phone and no one in sight. I had no option but to concentrate on mentally visualising a taxi coming towards me. After about five minutes, one came into view and I arrived in Bond Street with minutes to spare. The driver had no logical reason to be on the Heath. So did he respond to my thought on a subconscious level? I have always found that I get a response to my calls for help. Depending on the problem, help may come in the form of the written or spoken word, or someone else's actions, though it may be just the first step towards the solution. The main thing is to keep an open mind and remain on the alert so that signs are not missed.

Overcoming fear

I believe the memory of these incidents helped me to cope with Dennis who was not facing up to his problems. I had helped him financially and taken him to a series of doctors and psychiatrists, but to no avail. He was clearly slipping into a nervous breakdown, but unfortunately managed to fool the psychiatrist into believing that I was the source of the problem. Dr Weatherhead never took this problem as seriously as I hoped he would when I had sought his help unsuccessfully some years before. I quickly realised I had to take urgent action and to take full responsibility for my own life and family relationships which I had neglected, thinking it was my responsibility to help my friend. I acknowledged my mistake in allowing him to lean on me and that tough love was required to break the deadlock. More than once he physically transferred his frustrations and fears on to me by being violent (in addition to the more frequent mental violence) and in time I learned to overcome my fear of him by calmly putting to the test such phrases as 'perfect love casteth out fear.' I clearly remember one occasion when a sharp kitchen knife was aimed in my direction and with great control I emitted what I hoped was a strong feeling of goodwill. Amazingly, the knife was gradually withdrawn and he never attacked me again. From this moment on I had complete faith in positive thought. This experience helped me to understand that in dependency situations where both people have unresolved fears they transfer them to each other and when one of them retaliates it gives the other one permission to carry on the abuse. As I was able to present Dennis with a wall of goodwill his anger had to return to the source (himself).

Healing energy from a spiritual source

During this difficult period I received a form of spiritual healing in the form of a warm vibration moving down my spine during the night. I was definitely awake, but realised the healing was coming from a higher source. The healing removed all my previous feelings of resentment towards the man's mother whom I had wrongly blamed for most of his problems. In fact, I have never felt resentment of any kind since.

During my waking life, I became aware of extra strength from the higher source that continued to sustain me until I finally emerged from the relationship.

Meaningful recurring dreams

I also had two recurring dreams during this period, which I believe were my subconscious mind trying to tell me something. In one I found myself in an underground train only to realise I was travelling in the wrong direction. In the other, I was back in hospital (as a medical social worker) terrified because it was Monday when the ward sisters and I met to discuss the patients' welfare, and I had not bothered to interview a single patient. Finally, I realised my life was going in the wrong direction and that I was neglecting what I should be doing. The following is how I found the meaning in these dreams, which incidentally did not re-occur once I had acted upon their messages. The train dream, being simpler, was easier to understand. I was alerted by the horrible feeling that I was wasting my time travelling fast in the wrong direction and that I had to stop, get out of the train, catch another one back to where I had boarded it and start all over again. The journey was obviously the journey of life, the direction my purpose, and the train my relationship. I had not paid enough attention before committing myself to the relationship to realise that it would take me in the wrong direction. The hospital dream contained more symbolism and returned many times before I understood it fully. At first glance, it told me that I was neither preparing nor doing my work properly, leaving a lot undone. But it was the feeling of guilt the dream always left me with that caused me to take a second look, since in my waking life I did not feel guilty for having left medical social work. In the dream, I was working only in my office (restricted space) instead of venturing to the wards (wider world) to get to know the patients, their problems and medical conditions, and to help plan their aftercare in co-operation with the ward sisters (mother figures) and doctors (father figures). As all the main characters in a dream can relate to oneself I slowly realised it was a question of 'Physician heal thyself' to be followed by all sides of my nature, planning and preparing for more responsible work on a wider scale in the field of health and healing.

Taking full responsibility for my own life

I eventually issued Dennis with an ultimatum to take action within a certain period. He had not worked for sometime and I told him that he must either take a job, however simple, or take the advice of one of the good doctors who understood his situation, or else we would have to end our relationship. The days were running out and I knew he had taken no action. I had found a bed-sit in another part of London and had told my landlady that I planned to move. My sister, who hadn't been in touch for a while, suddenly asked me for the weekend and I was able to open up to her in a way I had never been able to do before. To my amazement she said 'Peter and I will come and help you move.' The night before I moved, I said goodnight to my friend who left at 10 pm, went to sleep for two hours, woke at midnight and quietly packed. It was during the time that the astronauts first landed on the moon (August 1969) and I could identify with them that night. In the morning, my sister and brother-in-law arrived earlier than planned. What a good thing they did because I later heard from my landlady, with whom I'd left a letter for Dennis, that he came round soon after we left, much earlier than usual (he lived nearby, but had a key). In deciding whether to issue the ultimatum I had to face the fact that he might commit suicide, which he had threatened to do more than once, and whether I would feel responsible if he did. I also knew his mother would almost certainly have blamed me. But, by then I had come to the firm belief that each one of us is on our own individual life path and here on earth to experience and learn from our own past mistakes. Above all, as adults, we are here to take full responsibility for our thoughts and actions. Friends and relatives can offer love and encouragement (as well as speaking the truth with goodwill) but are not here to live our life for us, which would only have a weakening effect. It is only by accepting responsibility for our own self-development that we become stronger.

In assuming too much responsibility for Dennis, I had unwittingly made it harder for him to find his own inner strength. At the same time I had neglected my own life path, family, friends and career and I felt sure it had become my duty to challenge him to work through his own problems and be responsible for the consequences of his own actions. It is my understanding that to do otherwise would be to hamper his soul's growth and that since I had left him with three people he already had confidence in and would stand by him, I felt that what happened subsequently was his responsibility, not mine. In my letter, which was intended to be a fair appraisal of our relationship, I had given him hope that we might be able to resume contact in six months or so if he took steps to deal with his problems. My action did shock him into finding employment, but during the following years, it was apparent that he had not dealt with his psychological problems because it never became possible to hold a normal conversation with him.

This intense relationship lasted for 12 years (1957–1969). It became clear to me that I was drawn into it by having too a great a need to be appreciated, and many people would say that I threw away the best years of my life. Whether I paid too high a price is difficult to answer. I needed an absorbing project to fill the void left by Jack's departure from my life and hadn't as yet found any degree of fulfilment in my work: teaching and therapy work still lay in the future. I emerged from this experience stronger in every way, having overcome some of my physical and character weaknesses. The lessons learned and the discovery of a totally satisfying philosophy was beyond price and for a long while I felt ahead of my contemporaries in life-learning skills. As my artist friend has commented more than once, 'In life we must always try to bring advantage out of disadvantage.'

Jack, knowing of my predicament, transferred money into a special bank account in New York in case I should have to run away. This was never necessary because I was confident that I had taken the right action for the right motives and had no fear of the consequences. Nevertheless, I shall remain eternally grateful to Jack for his generous offer of help.

Freedom to be my own person
I returned to Elizabeth Arden the following Monday. I had moved on the Saturday (2 August 1969), a date that I will never forget, and spent the weekend in the country with my sister and her family. They had tried to

persuade me to stay on for several days, but I was anxious to return to face whatever music awaited me. Business at Arden's boomed because all the clients wanted to know the next instalment of the drama that was unfolding! I knew I would be stalked, so warned the doorman at Arden's front entrance to ignore anyone with a plausible story who tried to gain access to me, which happened many times. For the first week, I took a taxi home each night and had already informed the police both in Bond Street and in St John's Wood of my predicament. Believe it or not, I was escorted up Bond Street each morning and in St John's Wood the police came to my rescue when I was finally tracked down. I was pestered almost daily with letters, phonecalls, meetings on buses, and intercepted on my way to and from work. None of this worried me because I didn't respond to Dennis in any way. It would have been impossible to hold a logical conversation because all he did was to react emotionally. He would even jump on and off buses to hold a conversation with me, but because I never replied, he had to answer his own questions in order to continue the conversation, much to the astonishment of the other passengers.

Later in 1969, I persuaded the manageress at Elizabeth Arden that it would be a good idea for me to work for a few weeks in the New York Salon in order to bring back new ideas for the London Salon that was shortly to move a few doors along Bond Street. It was an exciting few weeks. I received a warm welcome in New York and 'pretended' that I had emigrated because the artist was shortly to move permanently to the US with his family and hoped I would do the same. I experimented with the idea, but knew it would only work if my own life would develop better in the States because I could not be a part of his life. It could have worked. I loved New York, made friends and found a place to live. It was even possible that I might have been able to work in one or other of Miss Arden's health farms (Arizona and Maine). But in New York where I would be based, the work would have been quite regimented. In the US, I would be restricted by either what Miss Arden herself deemed I should do, or the head of the department, whereas in London I enjoyed the freedom, within limits, to do my own thing. In London, I was able to introduce yoga under the name of special relaxation exercises (this was in the early 1970s before yoga was universally accepted) and instituted health and fitness evening classes in the salon for air hostesses.

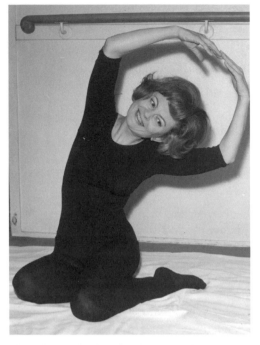

So, although I returned from America revitalised and bursting with new ideas, I realised London suited my independent nature better. Soon after my return from America, the artist and his family emigrated. On the day they sailed, I was massaging a favourite client and she said to me 'Mary, whatever is the matter with you today? The usual balance has gone out of your hands.' I know my mind was in turmoil and realised my feelings were being transferred through my hands. This proved to me that in any laying on of hands situation whether in therapeutic massage or spiritual healing, the essence can pass from one person to another. For any degree of benefit to take place it is therefore important that all therapists and healers alike remain in a state of emotional calm, so that they can be used as a channel through which healing energies can pass.

During this period I had a brief brush with Scientology. A client who was undergoing training with the organisation offered to 'clear' me (a form of psychoanalysis). I believe her offer was genuine, but I declined it as I feared being sucked into an organisation which I realised capitalised on people's vulnerability. Instead I read L. Ron. Hubbard's self-help book titled *Dianetics – The Modern Science of Mental Health* (latest publication 2007) which was surprisingly helpful.

Our individual links with universal energies from the moment of birth

Towards the end of 1971 I had managed to save up enough money for a deposit on a small flat and was lucky enough to find one in a nearby purpose-built block in St John's Wood. I had developed an interest in the effects of colour in decor and had enormous fun expressing my personality through my chosen colour schemes and furnishings. It was a totally satisfying experience. At this time I had just discovered another useful tool for self-help and understanding, Numerology, which is akin to Astrology, but easier to follow. It so happened that my flat number was 102 which reduces to 1+2=3. Briefly, Pythagoras the Greek mathematician developed his own theory that all life energies can be explained in numerical relationships. Energies generally associated with the number 3 are: artistic talent, ability for verbal or written self-expression, but may over-diversify and waste energies. It was in this flat that I would select and write the syllabus for the courses I would teach at the London College of Fashion from 1974–1983 and eventually write my 'magnum opus' that became self-work manuals for my clients.

At the same time I was studying the beneficial effects of colour, especially the visible light rays emitted by the sun (as seen in the rainbow) and discovering that all life on earth is linked to the movement and rhythms of Space that affect us all from the moment of birth.

The zodiac charts that follow indicate our links with specific colours, tissue salts and minerals also areas of our body that may need our attention.

Influence of the Sun on our organic make-up
In her book *Spectrobiology*, Maryla de Chrapowicki seeks to prove that as

we all draw our energy from the sun, in an ordered universe our health must surely be compared with the specific distribution of the sun's rays at the moment of birth. The Zodiac and Associated Energies Chart is intended as a guide to our organic make-up showing where weaknesses may lie, which elements and colours should predominate in the diet and how we may be affected by climate and atmospheric conditions.

The Zodiac is a region on the celestial sphere that extends to about 9° on each side of the ecliptic (the sun's apparent orbit) within which the Sun, Moon and Planets appear to move. It is divided into 12 equal sections, each measuring 30° of celestial longitude, bearing the names of the constellations that correspond to them (the signs of the Zodiac). The word Zodiac derives from the Greek words 'zoe' (life), 'diakos' (wheel) and 'zoon' (animal) – that is, the wheel of life and the circle of animals. In the womb, the embryo can be placed within the Zodiac circle – from Aries which rules the head, through Leo the heart, to Pisces the feet.

Seasonal and diurnal light changes

Due to the motion of the earth and its spherical surface, the sun's rays do not strike it evenly; in fact the proportion of the rays constantly changes from sunrise to sunset and from one season to another. The chart below indicates the predominant rays distributed to temperate zones throughout the year. Time used throughout is Greenwich Mean Time.

December to February		March to April		May to June	
Time	*Colour*	*Time*	*Colour*	*Time*	*Colour*
7–8 am	Ultra-violet / Purple	6–7 am	Ultra-violet / Purple	5–6 am	Ultra-violet
8–9 am	Violet	7–8 am	Violet	6–7 am	Purple
9–10 am	Indigo	8–9 am	Indigo	7–8 am	Violet
10–11 am	Blue	9–11 am	Blue	8–9 am	Indigo
11–12 am	Azure / Aquamarine	11–12 am	Azure / Aquamarine	9–10 am	Blue
12–1 pm	Turquoise	12–1 pm	Turquoise	10–11 am	Azure / Aquamarine
1–2 pm	Green	1–2 pm	Green	11–12 am	Turquoise
2–3 pm	Yellow	2–3 pm	Yellow	12–1 pm	Green
3–4 pm	Orange	3–4 pm	Orange	1–2 pm	Yellow
4 pm onwards	RSMIR	4 pm onwards	RSMIR	2–3 pm	Orange
				3–4 pm	Red
				4–5 pm	Scarlet
				5–6 pm	Magenta
				6–7 pm	Infrared

July to August		September to November	
Time	*Colour*	*Time*	*Colour*
4–5 am	Ultra-violet / Purple	5–6 am	Ultra-violet / Purple
5–6 am	Violet	6–7 am	Violet
6–8 am	Indigo	7–8 am	Indigo
8–9 am	Blue	8–9 am	Blue
9–10 am	Azure / Aquamarine	9–10 am	Azure / Aquamarine
10–11 am	Turquoise	10–11 am	Turquoise
11–12 am	Green	11–12 am	Green
12–2 pm	Yellow	12–1pm	Yellow
2–4 pm	Orange	1–2 pm	Orange
4 pm onwards	RSMIR	2 pm onwards	RSMIR

R = Red   S = Scarlet   M = Magenta   IR = Infrared

Zodiac and associated energies chart

Sun (Zodiac) sign	Ruling planet	Colour (indicates mood of the sign)	Bio-chemic tissue salt	Subdivision of sign	Constitutional centre	Elements and minerals	Colour energies
The Ram – Aries 21 Mar–20 Apr Element: Fire Mode: Cardinal Masculine energy type: Outgoing	**Mars** Symbolises vitality; influences the 5 senses, iron in the blood and sexual organs	Red	Kali Phos.	21–31 March 1–20 April	Hair and top of head Eyes, ears, nose	Nitrogen Oxygen Sulphur Magnesium Manganese	Indigo Blue
The Bull – Taurus 21 Apr–20 May Element: Earth Mode: Fixed Feminine energy type: Receptive	**Venus** Rules the throat and kidneys	Yellow (or pink or pale blue)	Nat. Sulph.	21–30 April 1–20 May	Cerebellum, nose, ears, mouth, neck Throat, larynx, lower jaw, tonsils, thyroid	Manganese Hydrogen Sodium	Blue Aqua-marine (or Azure)
The Twins – Gemini 21 May–20 June Element: Air Mode: Mutable Masculine energy type: Outgoing	**Mercury** Rules the respiratory system and sends brain signals to all parts of the nervous system	Violet (or lemon yellow)	Kali Mur.	21–31 May 1–20 June	Lungs, arms, shoulders, hands, and nerves Lungs, arms, shoulders, hands, muscles	Sodium Iron Copper Magnesium	Aqua-marine (or Azure Turquoise
The Crab – Cancer 21 June–20 July Element: Water Mode: Cardinal Feminine energy type: Receptive	**Moon** Rules breasts and stomach	Green	Cal. Fluor.	21–30 June 1–20 July	Breasts, stomach Thoracic spine, heart, elasticity of skin, and blood vessels	Magnesium Nitrogen Iron Sulphur	Turquoise Green
The Lion – Leo 21 July–21 Aug Element: Fire Mode: Fixed Masculine energy type: Outgoing	**Sun** Rules the heart; is the giver of life	Golden yellow / orange	Mag. Phos.	21–31 July 1–21 August	Heart, spinal column Small intestine, solar plexus, pancreas	Sulphur Copper Nitrogen Potassium Sodium	Greenish yellow (or lemon) Yellow
The Virgin – Virgo 22 Aug–22 Sept Element: Earth Mode: Mutable Feminine energy type: Receptive	**Mercury** Rules the respiratory system and sends brain signals to all parts of the nervous system	Purple, navy blue, brown	Kali Sulph.	22–31 August 1–22 Septr	Pancreas, solar plexus, large intestine Lumbar spine, large intestine, nervous system	Sodium Manganese	Yellow Orange

Sun (Zodiac) sign	Ruling planet	Colour (indicates mood of the sign)	Bio-chemic tissue salt	Subdivision of sign	Constitutional centre	Elements and minerals	Colour energies
The Scales – Libra 23 Sep–22 Oct Element: Air Mode: Cardinal Masculine energy type: Outgoing	**Venus** Rules the throat and kidneys	Yellow (or pink or pale blue)	Nat. Phos.	23–30 Sept 1–22 Oct	Adrenals, kidneys, lumbar spine Adrenals, kidneys, top of pelvis	Calcium Nitrogen Hydrogen	Orange Red
The Scorpion – Scorpio 23 Oct–21 Nov Element: Water Mode: Fixed Feminine energy type: Receptive	**Pluto** Rules the eliminatory system, reproduction and inner senses (clairvoyance, clairaudience)	Deep red	Cal. Sulph.	23–31 Oct 1–21 Nov	Bladder, descending colon, blood, reproductive organs Bladder, rectum, blood, reproductive organs	Hydrogen Calcium Calcium Oxygen Potassium	Red Scarlet
The Archer – Sagittarius 22 Nov – 20 Dec Element: Fire Mode: Mutable Masculine energy type: Outgoing	**Jupiter** Linked with the purifying function of the liver	Deep clear blue	Silica	22–30 Nov 1–20 Dec	Sacrum, rectum, thighs Sacrum, thighs	Potassium Fluorine Phosphorus	Scarlet Magenta
The Sea Goat – Capricorn 21 Dec–19 Jan Element: Earth Mode: Cardinal Feminine energy type: Receptive	**Saturn** Governs the skin and bony structure	White, black, dark green, brown	Cal. Phos.	21–31 Dec 1–19 Jan	Knees Knees, bones, joints, skin	Phosphorus Silicon Carbon	Magenta Purple
The Water Bearer – Aquarius 20 Jan–18 Feb Element: Air Mode: Fixed Masculine energy type: Outgoing	**Uranus** Related to the circulatory system	Uranium / electric blue	Nat. Mur.	20–31 Jan 1–18 Feb	Shins, ankles, venous and arterial circulation Shins, ankles, lymphatic circulation	Carbon Calcium Sulphur Iodine Iron	Purple Violet
The Fishes – Pisces 19 Feb–20 March Element: Water Mode: Mutable Feminine energy type: Receptive	**Neptune** Rules the lymphatic system	Soft azure blue, soft sea green, (aquamarine)	Ferr. Phos.	19–28 Feb 1–20 March	Feet, lymphatic system Feet, lymphatic system, mucous membranes	Iron Magnesium Nitrogen	Violet Indigo

Man is thought to have a strong affinity with the colour energies (visible light rays between the infrared and ultraviolet rays) emitted by the sun at the time of day and month of birth, and to radiate and use these freely throughout life. This could mean that we over-use them or that they are drawn upon subconsciously by those in need, so that we tend to become deficient in them. Therapists and healers may find they are best able to help conditions linked with the colour or element associated with their own personal sign (air, fire, water or earth). Equally, it is possible that we may lack not the main colour but the complementary colour associated with our opposite sign.

Any illness or weakness usually originates from the constitutional centre (the body area associated with the Zodiac sign), but more often will show up in the centre of the opposite sign. Two other likely areas are the centres midway between the birth sign and the opposite sign. Thus we should eat foods rich in the appropriate colour energies, elements and minerals, and supplement with tissue salts where necessary. Those of us born within a day or two of a change of sun sign (on the cusp) may also be affected by the influences of the adjacent sign.

All forms of energy involve action, reaction and interaction. In astrology, these qualities or modes are referred to as 'Cardinal', 'Fixed' and 'Mutable'. The Cardinal mode generates power, the Fixed concentrates power, and the Mutable distributes power. Each sun sign is associated with a specific mode and energy type described as either masculine (outgoing) or feminine (receptive). Each sun sign is also thought to be influenced by a specific planet.

Space does not allow for an exposé on colour therapy but here is the briefest of descriptions followed by a table that indicates how we can replenish our colour energies from the foods we eat.

Light (is energy, is colour) is life

> *The purest and most thoughtful minds*
> *Are those which love colour the most.*
> John Ruskin, *The Stones of Venice*

Colour therapy is a form of healing that uses visible light rays, those between ultraviolet and infrared first revealed in the middle of the 17th century by Isaac Newton when he split the spectrum. It is based on the assumption that everything on the planet is composed of energies from the sun's rays. These are measured in octaves of oscillatory frequencies made up of luminous electromagnetic particles transmuted into elements. An element is a substance such as silver, carbon or sulphur which cannot be split up into anything chemically. From these elements all matter including plants, animals and man is made. Many scientists, in particular G. P. Ghadiali have been able to establish a correlation between elements and colour although they are on different levels of vibrational frequencies.

Colour energies in relation to elements in foods

I have emphasised the element that is associated with a specific colour. Some elements appear under more than one colour heading because as well as the predominant colour they radiate several secondary colours.

Colour	Food	Elements
Red	Red-skinned apples, beetroot, red cabbage, cherries, redcurrants, red plums, radishes and raspberries	**Hydrogen**, iron, copper, potassium and zinc
Orange	Apricots, carrots, mangoes, cantaloupe melons, oranges, pumpkins, satsumas, swedes and tangerines	Carbon, iron, **calcium**, copper, selenium, manganese, zinc and silicon, slight association with oxygen
Yellow	Bananas, corn, egg yolks, grapefruit, lemons, honey-dew melons, parsnips, peaches, yellow peppers and pineapple	**Sodium**, **carbon**, phosphorus, calcium, zinc, chromium, copper, cobalt, manganese, magnesium and molybdenum
Green	Green-skinned apples, avocados, beans, green cabbage, courgettes, cucumber, green gooseberries, green-skinned grapes, green vegetable greens, kiwi fruit, lettuce, peas, green peppers and spinach	Carbon, **nitrogen**, sodium, copper, chromium, cobalt and **chlorine**
Blue	Blueberries, damsons, blue grapes, blue plums	**Oxygen**, cobalt, copper, zinc and manganese

Indigo	See under blue and violet	Associated with oxygen, chromium, iron, and copper
Violet	Aubergines, blackberries, purple grapes, and purple vegetable greens	Iron, manganese, calcium and **cobalt**
Magenta	See under red	**Potassium**
Lemon	Similar to those under yellow, in particular lemons and grapefruit	**Iodine**, **iron**, phosphorus and **sulphur**
Turquoise	See under blue and green	Chromium, **fluorine** and zinc
Scarlet	See under red	**Manganese**

Here is a brief introduction to numerology that has proved useful for clients and friends.

Numerology, the science of numbers

The 24-hour day, the intervals of night and day, the seven days of the week, the lunar and calendar months, and the 'Ages' of the Zodiac are all discrete units of time that astrological scientists have been at pains to understand for centuries.

The 'great year' is the period of approximately 25,920 years that the earth takes to pass through the influence of each of the signs of the Zodiac in turn. At the vernal equinox (around 20/21 March when the sun passes over the Equator, and night and day are equal in length), the constellation of stars lying behind the sun changes slightly. This is due to a slight wobble in the earth's rotation, caused by the sun's own orbital movement. According to astrological scientists, this exerts influences upon the earth, in accordance with the specific Zodiac sign the constellation represents, and is thought to provide mankind with opportunities to evolve to a higher level of living.

During the course of 25,920 years, the earth's polar axis describes a full circle. It takes 2160 years for the earth to pass through each sign (25,920 divided by 12 = 2160, the period of a 'great month'). A 'great day' (25,920 divided by 365) is 71 years, hence the biblical reference to man's life span being three score years and ten.

The birth of Christ heralded the beginning of the 'Piscean Age' and soon after the turn of the 21st century the earth will come under the influence of Aquarius. Throughout history, tremendous upheavals (often foretold by prophets and soothsayers) have accompanied the approach of a new age and this one is no exception. It has been forecast that if we can let go our attachment to material things and learn to live by spiritual values, a new golden age of brotherhood could dawn upon the earth.

Associated with these divisions of time are the seven basic colours, the seven basic tones in the musical scale, the nine planets and the basic numbers 1–9. The ancient civilisations, Chaldeans, Hindus, Hebrews and Egyptians all had their own system of tabulating the laws governing the movements in space and the way they affect everything on the planet, including humankind. They believed in the link between numbers, letters and colours. Pythagoras, the Greek philosopher and mathematician, who lived around the 6th century BC, studied this ancient science and developed his own theory that all life can be explained in numerical relationships. The Sanskrit teachers acknowledged that planetary cycles affect us all, and many people feel that life works much better if we recognise tidal rhythms in ourselves, and learn to flow with them.

To numerologists, those who study the science of numbers, the birth date is the most significant number, as it is to astrologists. This is because the birth date is unalterable. There may be numerical vibrations associated with the letters (according to the number each letter represents) in our name and address or in our 'phone number, but all these are changeable. Our names change, by abbreviation, by nick-names, and when a woman's surname changes through marriage. To find your birth number based on your birth date, write down the relevant digits, then add up the day, month and year separately, reduce each section to a single digit, or an 11 or 22 – known as master numbers. Then add these sections together, finally reducing them to a single digit, or an 11 or 22. This is called the destiny number. It indicates the main lessons to be learned in the life and the type of opportunities that will be available for this purpose.

To give an example, take the birth date 22.8.1982:

22 for the day, **8** by itself represents the month,
$1 + 9 + 8 + 2 = 20 = 2 + 0 = 2$ for the year.
$22 + 8 + 2 = 32 = 3 + 2 = 5$ is the destiny number.

Although the destiny number will exert the strongest influence on the life, the digit(s) representing the day, month and year each contain a sub-lesson. The day refers to the individual personal aspects, the harmonic note and what is needed for the life to blossom. The month refers to more general matters and to the middle years. The year relates to the undercurrents of events and to what can be achieved in later years.

The significance of double numbers

When working out your destiny number and working with the numbers that represent the day, month and year of your birth, you should be aware that some double digit numbers have special significance. The day of your birth may be 11, 13, 14, 16, 19 or 22, for instance, all of which are significant double numbers. Your birth month may be 11 (November) and the year of your birth may also add up to a significant double number. The years 1918 and 1984, for instance, add up to 19 and 22 respectively.

Numbers 11 and 22 are master numbers and deal with idealism. People born under the influence of these numbers are given opportunities to put their ideals into practice. Whether they choose to live up to their full potential is, of course, up to them; they may choose instead to work with the numbers in their single digit forms: $11 = 2$, or $22 = 4$.

The numbers 13, 14, 16 and 19 are signs that there are problems arising from mistakes made in the past (for those with a belief in reincarnation, perhaps in a past life). For instance, in the case of 19, this indicates that both 1 and 9 energies have been misused; but the most important lessons will lie along the path of the number in its single digit form, in this case 1. In the current life, the individual concerned will exhibit the negative traits of the number 1; he/she will be exposed to the negative effects of the previous energy misuse and will have to overcome these effects (without feeling victimised), before being able to realise the positive potential of 1. Energy misuse might mean that the person had previously abused power by dominating others (negative 1) to fulfil selfish desires (negative 9), or had been too reliant on others (negative 1). In the current life, he/she may feel dominated or restricted by others, fear rejection and suffer shyness.

That person will have to learn to stand on his/her own feet and have the courage of his/her convictions, bearing in mind that other people have needs too, and neither dominating nor being dominated by other people.

If the significant number occurs in the day of birth, the obstacles that must be overcome in order to use the energies correctly will occur in the early years. Significant numbers that occur as the destiny number mean that the influences will be experienced to a greater degree and throughout life, but will naturally present fewer problems if the lesson is mastered early in life.

Whatever your birth date, you will now have a set of numbers to work with.

Basic qualities and indications of the number
1　Individuality, courage, strong beliefs, ability for leadership and to pioneer new concepts (often thought too avant-garde by others), sense of responsibility, sometimes intolerance, ambition, strong ego, forcefulness often mistaken for obstinacy, loyalty to a cause; loving in nature, a hard worker yet demanding; a liking for movement, physical and mental, otherwise likely to become bored.
　　Main lesson – self-reliance, leadership without being self-centred or dominating.
2　Tact, adaptability, gentleness, need for harmonious relationships; may be easily upset and want peace at any price, which leads to being put upon, self-pity and frustration; a warm, sympathetic nature at home in the caring professions; love and loyalty for family including love of animals; sense of rhythm as applied to music, dance and poetry; difficulty in making decisions; need for a firm partner; makes a reliable colleague.
　　Main lesson – co-operation with others; learning the art of peaceful persuasion neither using force nor becoming a 'door-mat'.

3   A magnetic, charming personality; sociability often with social ambition, intelligent thinker; resilience, versatility, enthusiasm, facility with words and ability to motivate people; a love of colour, jewellery and fashion; artistic talent (painting, music, acting), showmanship; views life as an art form and a stage; strong intuition, but tendency to do too many things at once and suffer impatience and nervous tension, or become involved in gossip, trivia and extravagance.
Main lesson – expansive self-expression without boastfulness or being too critical of others.

4   Willingness to work hard; down-to-earth qualities, efficiency and organising ability; strong will; sense of loyalty and responsibility especially to family and friends; if negative, may have a love-hate relationship for routine and be too rigid or blunt in speech or attitude; ability to build a family or business; need for a regular, balanced life and a dependable partner; dislike of all superficiality and pretension.
Main lesson – practical organisation, learning to work hard and constructively with limiting circumstances, without being stubborn or careless over details.

5   A quick, lively mind and the need to seek truth; adaptability; many varied talents, artistic abilities – centred on production, for example commercial artist, producer, author, composer, manager of art gallery or antique business; enthusiastic communicator, so could be a gifted teacher; a liking for variety and travel; tendency to be restless and to scatter energies in too many directions, or become self-indulgent and indiscreet; needs stable associates.
Main lesson – to experience widely and wisely, undergo many changes and use freedom constructively without hurting others or becoming a 'rolling stone'.

6   Whereas 5 tends to be untidy, 6 is neat; has practical, creative and domestic abilities, strong sense of responsibility, liking for routine; suitability for secretarial or executive rather than managerial position; methodical nature, conservative, careful with money, diplomatic, but could appear narrow-minded and over-protective in attitude; usually loving, caring and generous; a flair for beauty and colour and need for harmony in surroundings and relationships.

Main lesson – responsibility, tact, caring for others with an unselfish (not possessive) love.

7   Great sensitivity and interest in discovering scientific, psychic and spiritual meaning of life; need to spend a lot of time alone to analyse, research and develop insight; creativity and potential for becoming an artist, philosopher or educator, but has strong emotions and need for constant movement and excitement which can lead to extreme mood swings, aloofness, too much introspection and unwise decisions; a loveable nature and entertaining company.

Main lesson – mental analysis, wisdom; learning to recognise illusion; develop innate skills and find answers to problems alone, without fearing loneliness or failure.

8   Ambitious for success, power and wealth incorporating likelihood of becoming a skilled administrator and good arbitrator, exercising balanced judgement and managing financial affairs efficiently; logical, practical, usually truthful, but dogmatic with a tendency to be ponderous and intolerant; may make the mistake of acquiring wealth and material comforts as ends in themselves and not receive the pleasure expected. In contrast, has compassion and feelings of tenderness for those in trouble, including animals, but may find difficulty in expressing deep feelings to loved ones; potential (seldom realised) for recognising that material freedom can mean relying very little on money or material things for happiness.

Main lesson – the mental satisfaction, power and freedom that come from hard work and using success for the benefit of the community without misusing money or power.

9   A universal attitude; sense of adventure, need to travel to avoid restlessness; need to work for benefit-of-all; broad-mindedness, generosity, compassion, creative ability, humanitarianism, and personal ambition - which could cause inner conflict; potential for inspiring others as a teacher, counsellor, artist or leader of a humanitarian organisation, but may have to develop patience and persistence.

Main lesson – selfless service to mankind on a wide front, without prejudice, not expecting anything in return but finding that love and friendship are received and other personal needs satisfied as a result of serving others.

11 Intuitive and psychic abilities with a tendency to drift through life day-dreaming or to experience dissatisfaction from using the power for selfish ends; analytical mind but can allow reason to suppress intuition instead of following up hunches in a practical manner; innate sense of balance and ability to create harmony between conflicting points of view; a love of art, music, beauty; potential for becoming a painter, composer, dancer or a visionary and enlightened spiritual advisor.

Main lesson – to develop intuition and spiritual awareness in order to inspire and illuminate others by example, without remaining an impractical dreamer or being concerned with material needs.

13 (1 + 3 = 4) implies the need to use the will constructively to complete all rightful tasks instead of leaving them half-done or pushing them on to others.

14 (1 + 4 = 5) implies the need to use freedom constructively; includes the warning not to use thought and speech in destructive criticism or to become a 'rolling stone', or to give in to self-indulgence.

16 (1 + 6 = 7) There is a need to be aware of illusion and to distinguish it from real inspiration. There is also the need to avoid hurting others in a loving relationship; need to go on in the face of any disappointment or failure and to find its cause.

19 (1 + 9 = 10 = 1 + 0 = 1) teaches that we get from life the measure of what we put into it so that those who complain that life passes them by must learn to accept responsibility, become self-reliant (learning that independence must not be confused with dominance) and willing to serve mankind. Only by doing so will life take on meaning.

22 Combines the idealism of 11 with the capacity to visualise a master plan and to realise ideals in a practical form – for example, as part of a healing organisation; should avoid the tendency to become 'lost' in details that could be dealt with by others. Exceptional capabilities and charisma, often using unorthodox methods; tends to suffer from nervous tension in coping with powerful inner forces; can fear failure and be overwhelmed by the awesome potential, or use the power ruthlessly for selfish ends.

Main lesson – to use practical gifts and spiritual vision to benefit mankind on a large scale, often having to overcome vast obstacles, without succumbing to fear or being concerned with accumulating personal wealth.

The number value of letters

1	2	3	4	5	6	7	8	9
A	B	C	D	E	F	G	H	I
J	K	L	M	N	O	P	Q	R
S	T	U	V	W	X	Y	Z	

Applying your knowledge of numerology
In order to show you how to use this information for increased understanding of yourself and others, I have included the very briefest analysis of my birth date – 19.3.1927.

My birth date:
19 – personal aspects/harmonic note/requirements for life
$1 + 9 = 10 = 1 + 0 = 1$
March = **3** – general matters/middle years
1927 – current of destiny/what can be achieved
$1927 = 19 = 1 + 9 = 10 = 1 + 0 = 1$

Added together, $1 + 3 + 1 = 5$ = main path of destiny or life lesson. My main path of destiny therefore is along the vibration of 5.

Since the number 5 indicates that I have to learn to use freedom constructively, this suggests that I will have many opportunities to experience widely and make wiser choices. It may explain why I have gradually moved from 'secure' situations to find fulfilment in jobs where I am self-employed. But I must avoid scattering my energies in too many directions, and be prepared to let go outworn views and activities.

While the lesson remains throughout the life, each year has its own lesson number although this remains secondary to the life lesson. The lesson for each year can be found by adding the birthday, the birth month and the current year in question, for example:

$$
\begin{array}{ccc}
\textit{19} & \textit{3} & \textit{1985} \\
1 + 9 = 10 = 1 + 0 = \mathbf{1} & \mathbf{3} & 1 + 9 + 8 + 5 = 23 = 2 + 3 = \mathbf{5} \\
1 \quad + \quad 3 \quad + & & 5 \qquad \qquad = \mathbf{9}
\end{array}
$$

Therefore 9 was my secondary lesson for 1985.

Every nine years, when you apply the day and month of your birthday to the current year, you will again have a number that reduces to the same digit(s) as your destiny number. In my case I had to wait until 1999 – and again in 2008 when the 19.03.1999/ 19.03.2008 – which reduced to 5, my original destiny number. This nine year cycle can be regarded as a culmination and the beginning of a new cycle of opportunities.

The number 19 is assessed as '19' as well as 1. Nineteen occurs in my birth year as well as in my birthday and implies a special lesson, previously described. For the implication of 3 (my birth month), see indications and qualities of the number 3.

I believe we 'choose' our parents and date of birth in order that our environment provides the best opportunities for learning whatever lessons we have come here to learn. I also believe that our parents, providing they are on the right wavelength, are intuitively 'told' what name to give us so that the numerical energies associated with the letters give us the characteristics we need to fulfil our potential.

The whole name reduced to a single digit or master number (11 or 22) is called the expression number. It represents the potential of all our natural abilities and the manner in which we express them, as in a vocation or career, hobbies and home life.

The expression number is found by adding the number values of the letter in each name separately, reducing each name to a single digit or master number, and noting if a karmic number (13, 14, 16 or 19) is revealed. Then is the sum of all the names added together and the total reduced to a single digit or master number.

Although many of us ignore our middle name(s), or use an abbreviation of our first name, or a nickname, and a woman changes her surname when she marries, the full name given at birth is the one used for basic analysis. Any other variations can then be assessed for their modifying effects.

A brief analysis of my own name is as follows:

M	4		
A	1	}	21 = 2 + 1 = 3
R	9		
Y	7		

W	5		
I	9		
N	5	}	32 = 3 + 2 = 5
T	2		
O	6		
N	5		

P	7		
E	5		
R	9		
I	9	}	48 = 12 = 1 + 2 = 3
G	7		
O	6		
E	5		
			Total: 3 + 5 + 3 = 11

So my expression number is 11. This indicates that I have psychic abilities and a sympathetic nature, which may have led me into social work and later to take up natural and spiritual therapies. It is difficult to live up to the challenges of a master number and I can see all too clearly how some of my earlier mistakes were due to the negative aspects of 11 and its lower form, 2. I used to get easily upset and live on my nerves. I tended to day-dream and allow reason to suppress hunches, until I learned from emotionally painful experiences the perils of ignoring intuition.

It is important to remember that just as positions of the Zodiac signs and planets in our astrological charts provide us with the best 'tools' for accomplishing our life's tasks, so do our numerological patterns. The symbols are different but the message is the same, and there is no such thing as 'good' or 'bad' patterns. Our individual patterns represent our potential for maximum development, but the degree to which we fulfil our potential depends upon how much we use our free will to work with the positive aspects.

If you find it strange that a name should have vibrations that can truly indicate our personality or life trends, try saying a name and listening to its rhythm or atmosphere and what effects the consonants and vowels create. You must be instinctive with your reactions otherwise you will start to think of all the friends you have with this particular name and try to make it fit their personality. Try it: George, for instance, sounds a down to earth person, round and warm, even if not in actual physique! Elisabeth has four syllables suggesting solidarity, firmness, reliability, but with a light touch – especially if spelt with an 's'. Although I have only scratched the surface of this fascinating subject, I hope I have stimulated you to find out more for yourself.

Branching out – new beginnings

To continue with the narrative, the same year that I moved to my flat, 1971, a producer and director from the BBC came to see me asking if I could recommend anyone suitable to teach exercises to women in their planned keep-fit series, as part of their Continuing Education department. I gave them several names; one in particular was Lotte Berk, famous in her day for her enthusiastic, but sometimes over-vigorous, routines that led to 'victims' tottering down to Bond Street for me to pick up the pieces. Much to my surprise I was called to an audition at the Television Centre which caused the Elizabeth Arden publicity machine to go into overdrive. I had to have my hair and make-up professionally done and off I went. Before the day dawned the nervous anticipation caused me to lose weight and I experienced feelings of euphoria, warning me of the danger of slipping into the attitude that food was unnecessary (akin to anorexia). So I took immediate steps to re-engage with food and felt uplifted on to another wavelength (beyond nerves) similar to the experience in the pulpit some years earlier. A few weeks later I heard that the BBC had offered me the role, but because of programme scheduling the series would not be made for at least a year. The first Cranks Health Food Shop and restaurant opened in the centre of London at this time and several of us in the department organised a weekly delivery of the most delicious homemade yoghurts I've ever tasted, before or since. I also continued to study all aspects of whole health including the benefits of vitamin and mineral supplements.

If you live in a town and are not lucky enough to grow your own fruit and vegetables, I recommend naturally produced vitamin and mineral supplements (medically proved more effective than those produced synthetically); it's helpful to take them if you are following a self-improvement programme, during the winter or when you are unable to obtain sufficient fresh foods, and at other times according to need, such as when under stress or sick.

However, those of you who lead a rigorous city life, as I do, exposed to constant air pollution and having to rely upon café-style snacks for lunch, will benefit from taking supplements (in appropriate amounts) all year round. Since doing so myself, I have experienced a marked increase in energy and resistance to common ailments.

Depending upon our current level of health and aspirations to improve it, as a rough guide these supplements should include vitamin A 5,000–7,500 iu, 25–75 mg., each of the five major B vitamins (B1, B2, B3, pantothenic acid and B6), vitamin C 1,000–3,000 mg., vitamin D 400 iu, vitamin E (d-alpha tocopherol) 100–500 iu – according to medical advice in the case of heart problems, calcium 150 mg., magnesium 100 mg., iron 10–15 mg., zinc 10–17 mg., manganese 2.5–6 mg., chromium 20–100 mcg., selenium 25–50 mcg.

It is important not to take large doses of isolated B vitamins in pill form since this can cause an imbalance amongst the rest of the B complex vitamins.

Since most minerals are not absorbable in their pure state, in order to maximise absorption they are bound with another substance to make, for example, zinc gluconate. To ensure your supplements provide the amounts listed above, it is important to distinguish between the dosage of the mineral plus binder and the mineral itself. For example, a supplement advertised as zinc gluconate 50 mg. will probably contain 5 mg. of pure zinc. Nowadays, most minerals also state the actual amount of the mineral on the label e.g. zinc gluconate 50 mg. (5 mg. zn.).

I had been using biochemic tissue salts for some time and began introducing them to interested clients along with general dietary advice. At this time I had also persuaded Elizabeth Arden to allow me to have private lessons with Beatrice Conway who had trained with a renowned India guru. She had gained a reputation for teaching Hatha Yoga (a contemplative form of exercise) at two popular health farms in the south of England and it was my intention after completing the training to introduce it to my clients as special relaxation exercises as it would be at least another decade before yoga became acceptable to the general population. Ava Gardiner, in particular, became a great devotee of these exercises. I found the emphasis on balanced breathing (an even in and out breath) helped me to sustain my energy for longer periods without swinging from over-activity to exhaustion. Energy is to a large extent self-generating if used in a balanced way (positively and evenly) with a period of activity followed by a pause. By easing carefully into the posture (never straining nor giving up too soon) it becomes easier to recognise how we contribute to our body's discomfort by tightening muscles and joints too strongly in response to nervous tension or by lifting or carrying weights incorrectly and so on. We can then alter our behaviour and react more gently so as to prevent a recurrence. Used conscientiously, yoga can be a useful tool both for self-understanding and self-help. Quite apart from the obvious benefits of improved posture, increased flexibility, muscle strength and more efficient breathing, yoga fosters a positive mental outlook by the letting go of a negative attitude and can aid such internal functions as digestion and elimination.

Later I took extra training from B.K.S. Iyengar, considered by many to be the father of present-day yoga. I regard his books as yoga 'bibles' but was horrified to witness him pushing some of his 'disciples' into extreme positions, even reducing them to tears which I thought was physically dangerous and not in tune with the spirit of yoga.

Here is a brief explanation of the meaning of yoga to show that it is not as obscure as its language may suggest. Yoga is one of six orthodox systems of Indian philosophy and its language is Sanskrit, a branch of Hindi. The name is derived from a Sanskrit word 'yui' meaning to 'join' or to 'yoke' and the Latin word 'yugum' meaning 'union'. In other words, the practice of yoga provides an opportunity to bring all parts of our nature into a state of harmony and link our energies with those of Spirit / the Source. As with other religions and philosophies, yoga recognises a trinity teaching that God, the Universal Source represents the 'Father / Mother' principle and the part of God (nature) that exists in the Universe represents the Child element. At a more earthly level, yogis recognise another trinity: mind, vitality or energy force known as Prana, and matter, all of which descend from Spirit in that order. So as Einstein once put it, it is as if God 'thought' and then sent forth energies to form the universe.

Prana is found in both nature and in the human body. It is believed that at birth we have our own individual supply that is stored in the base of the spine. In addition, we take it in through fresh, unpolluted air, spring or spa waters, and fresh unprocessed raw food. Prana is thought to travel through the spine and collect at energy wheels (centres) called chakras situated near gland and nerve centres from which it both circulates to the rest of the body and emanates from the body to form an atmosphere of vibrations known as the aura.

The aura

According to mystics, the aura includes emotional, psychic and even spiritual radiation and acts as a subtle, protective 'envelope'. The presence of the aura was discovered in the early 19th century by Franz Mesmer who taught that the stream of cosmic energies coming via the sun and beyond are drawn into the spiritual part of the aura as white light, then distributed to the rest of the body and broken down into the vibrations of the visible light rays (between the ultraviolet and infrared rays namely: violet, indigo, blue, green, yellow, orange and red), each of the vibrations going to the appropriate energy centre (chakra). There are seven main chakras and each vibrates in accordance with and radiates its own particular colour: violet (crown centre), indigo (brow), blue (throat), green (heart), yellow (solar plexus), orange (spleen/sacrum), and red (base of spine). If white light being drawn into the body is blocked for any reason by strong fear, resentment or hatred for instance, the endocrine glands will be thrown out of balance and physical illness will occur. This causes a corresponding dip in the aura and a change in the colour radiation. The chakras act as alchemists, transforming thoughts, the elements, colour, sound and food into mental and physical stamina, balance and spiritual attainment. White light or vital force enters the body in the air we breathe and in pure water and unadulterated food.

Space does not allow a description of postures here, but I hope this brief introduction will inspire readers to seek out a reputable Hatha Yoga class. Although the language of yoga is different, the essence of yoga does not conflict with my own philosophy and therapies, (colour therapy, reflexology, numerology and biochemic tissue salts) all of which are representative of the Oneness of the Universe.

AURA AND CHAKRA ENERGIES OF A FULLY EVOLVED HEALTHY PERSON

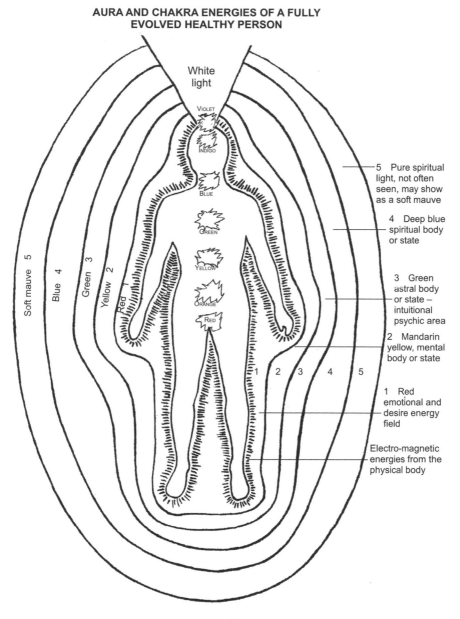

White light

VIOLET

INDIGO

BLUE

GREEN

YELLOW

ORANGE

RED

Soft mauve 5

Blue 4

Green 3

Yellow 2

Red 1

5 Pure spiritual light, not often seen, may show as a soft mauve

4 Deep blue spiritual body or state

3 Green astral body or state – intuitional psychic area

2 Mandarin yellow, mental body or state

1 Red emotional and desire energy field

Electro-magnetic energies from the physical body

Moving on

During my latter days at Elizabeth Arden, possibly precipitated by the Princess Margaret incident, the manageress confessed they were working me too hard and perhaps I had better find an easier job, possibly in management. I found a job in management, but it was not easier. For some reason I have always worked progressively harder with each new job!

I left Elizabeth Arden (May 1972) to run the health complex at the newly re-built Berkeley Hotel in Knightsbridge. It would involve very long hours as I needed to spend the evenings purchasing stock and choosing staff and so on, while working out my notice at Elizabeth Arden in the day time.

At the Berkeley Hotel, the complex consisted of an open-air swimming pool with a sun roof, and a sauna and massage department on the floor below. I was directly responsible to the General Manager of the hotel, a highly efficient and charismatic Italian. The overall boss was Sir Hugh Wontner, Chairman of the Savoy group of hotels (soon to become Lord Mayor of the City of London). I remember my interview when he bore down on me from a great height (he was well over six feet to my mere five feet) and said with an explanatory gesture, 'I think if someone tried to push you down, you'd bounce straight up again, like a jack in the box.' My one regret was that the hotel swimming pool was to be opened two weeks before the rest of the department, which I knew would undermine my authority with the pool attendants and bar staff – as it did for a while. Apart from this I had very few problems, except for a male masseur who disliked having a female boss and tried to stir things up from time to time. In the end he exposed himself as having lied about a serious incident so gave me cause to sack him. During my time at the hotel I had occasion to get angry at times and was pleased to find that I had not forgotten the lesson I had learned from previous times with Dennis, when I overcame my fear of emotional confrontation and was able to keep complete logical control.

A karmic relationship

A few weeks before I was due to leave Elizabeth Arden, a psychic told me that I would meet an important man there. Sure enough I did, but for some time I thought he was quite objectionable. On the surface he was a pushy, impatient, immaculately dressed larger than life character whose behaviour challenged me on all fronts; the last thing I needed at the time. He appeared to be a successful well-travelled entrepreneurial businessman with all the accoutrements including a Rolls Royce, which failed to impress me. Later he was to tease me saying I was a poor judge of character. He often stayed at the hotel and was one of the first guests to visit our department. I had decided not to give treatments myself so that any available tips went to my staff, giving me more time to supervise. But he was intent on having a massage from the manageress (he would say he had good taste and always demanded the best!). He would even request a warm towelling robe, slippers and towel to be delivered to his room, prior to coming to the department. I firmly, but politely refused his request as no equipment was to leave our department, these battles were repeated on a regular basis. Later on I discovered that the entire hotel had heard about the bossy woman who ruled her department with a rod of iron. In a similar vein I had earned a reputation at Arden's that followed me to the Berkeley for having a will of iron with a gentle manner and (as a masseuse) having iron fingers, but gentle hands. Two sides to my nature that I needed to keep in balance. However, I was eventually tricked into treating him. I had decided the job required me to work unsociable hours to begin with, 8 am–12 noon and 4–8 pm and one morning the inevitable happened. The pushy man, Duncan, wanted a massage very early and I was the only one on duty so couldn't refuse. Much to my annoyance, I found we had a lot in common and eventually discovered a sensitive, artistic and very private soul underneath the often brash exterior. In contrast to his working life and one of the few ways he could relax, he had taught himself to paint in oils. He developed different styles and was able to sell his work very successfully when he fell on hard times later in his life. His deep love of the countryside and passion for the sea (he had run away to serve in the Royal Navy in World War II) always figured in his imaginative paintings, some of which adorn my walls and have become my most treasured possessions.

Before he became a friend, he managed to find my home phone number and one Sunday evening rang me for a chat. Next day he said he hoped he hadn't disturbed me, but did enjoy talking to me. At the time he was face down on the massage table and to my horror I heard myself saying 'Of course you didn't disturb me. You are my dearest friend and can call me any time of day or night.' I was mortified and had no idea where the words came from ... they must have come from the depths of my soul. He was not a free man so nothing could come of our friendship, but we developed a strong bond of understanding and trust which, in spite of periods when we lost contact, lasted for over thirty years. I became convinced that we were soulmates and had known each other in a past life. Had I not overcome my emotional neediness during the Dennis relationship I am sure I could not have enjoyed such a good relationship with Duncan in which neither of us needed to make emotional demands on the other. We were able to enjoy the ebb and flow and natural interaction where each of us was free to be his or her own person.

Study courses in spiritual psychotherapy

During my first few months at the Berkeley I was introduced to the College of Spiritual Psychotherapeutics in Kent, and had a consultation with the principal, Ronald Beasley. He understood immediately the problems I had passed through and lessons learned, without me having to tell him anything. He said I would benefit from his residential courses, part one of which was due to take place in November of that year. There were 25 people ahead of me on the waiting list, but he seemed sure I would eventually be offered a place, which did happen. I had not been at the hotel long enough to be eligible for leave, paid or unpaid, but I explained to the manager the importance of the course to me though not expecting him to appreciate the contents. Very few people were open to esoteric philosophy in the 1970s and I emphasised that my loyalty was to the hotel and was totally prepared to forgo the course if it jeopardised my job. He kept me on tenterhooks almost up to the last minute and then said I could have paid leave. In retrospect I think he was teasing me by making out it was a difficult decision for him.

The first course was a mind-blowing experience. It was such a welcome change to meet people with similar beliefs and I often felt like jumping for joy in the lectures. We became a closely knit group, ate vegetarian food and only left the centre once to visit the Rudolf Steiner Centre in London. It became clear that we were finding it difficult to adjust to the outside world, having been in a rarefied atmosphere, because when we went for a walk we collapsed in uncontrollable giggles for no apparent reason. After two weeks when I finally returned to the Berkeley, I felt I'd been on another planet and it was with great self-control that I brought myself down to earth, helped by the discovery that owing to my staff's carelessness there had been a small fire in the department in my absence.

Over the next few years I attended the complete series of progressive courses at the college. We were introduced to all aspects of esoteric philosophy and healing, which included a spiritual overview of every level of life found in Nature (rocks, insects, flowers, fish, animals and humans), also aspects of less familiar belief systems such as Ancient Wisdom, Theosophy, Spiritualism, Buddhism and Yoga philosophy all of which believe in the Oneness of Nature. We learned about the Universal Laws such as Cause and Effect, Reincarnation and Karma and the courses gave structure to these beliefs and helped us appreciate our relationship with the rhythms and forces of nature. We were also introduced to the various levels of development in our own system, from survival instincts, appetites, creative energies, emotions, mental, psychic, and spiritual energies. In the practical training we learned specific massage and counselling techniques all with an added spiritual dimension, as well as a form of chakra energy balancing (akin to yoga) similar to Reiki healing, but requiring a higher degree of personal development to be fully effective. The college also had an individual approach to colour healing and reflexology, in both of which I had received training elsewhere.

'Don't just sit there' television series
To return to the narrative, in the spring of 1973, BBC Television announced that our series would begin in April for ten weeks. It was called 'Don't just sit there' and was the last BBC programme to be made in black and white. The hotel was pleased to give me time off to do this, hoping that any publicity would wash off on them. But as the BBC had met me at Elizabeth Arden they wouldn't agree to the hotel's name appearing on the credits.

There were three main contributors to the programme: Alan Howard, a doctor who was to talk about nutrition, Al Murray, a male gymnastics teacher, and myself. Al was to teach exercises to Willie Rushton, a well known satirical writer and actor, although the producer had wanted Terry Wogan, an up and coming radio DJ at the time, but he wasn't free. I taught exercises to Julie Stevens, a very friendly girl who was a presenter on Children's TV programmes.

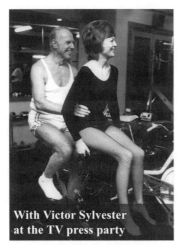

With Victor Sylvester at the TV press party

Willie was an ideal choice, very funny, but a reluctant exerciser and dieter; someone the viewers could identify with. Fortunately he managed to lose some weight and improve his shape during the series much to the relief of Al Murray who didn't think he was as keen as he should have been. Willie was particularly kind to me. I was the only one who had never done television before and he put me at my ease by saying I was a natural (I just hope he meant it!). The producer and director couldn't have been more helpful and we three contributors provided the material for our own section in the book that became part of the series and was reprinted many times.

Before the series began the producer took me aside and said, 'Mary there's one thing that worries me. You speak so quickly.' She and the director tried to rehearse me at a slower pace which didn't work very well, but I assured them that when I was in teaching mode I would speak very slowly and that is what happened.

The first recording went incredibly smoothly. I remember waiting in the wings to go on set and actually heard myself breathing slowly and deeply in a yoga manner (this must have happened at a subconscious level, I did not initiate it consciously). At the same time, I felt raised up into another dimension where nerves did not exist. Maybe it was my guardian angel or members of my family, like my father, sending me extra help. My one mistake was to look at the wrong camera just once during the recording, which can give the impression of nerves. When the programme was transmitted one of my male masseurs, Billy, the one who had resented having a female boss, was quick to tell me that I looked nervous. That cured me of looking at wrong cameras!

I watched the first transmission with my family in Sussex: mother, sister and brother-in-law and two nieces. My younger niece (aged 7 at the time) was transfixed and was heard boasting to her friends that her aunt was on TV. Fortunately, the programmes were well received.

The following year, 1974, the series was repeated and during that summer I went on a tour of the Holy Land, Jordan and Israel, with the Principal and a group from the College of Spiritual Psychotherapeutics. We went to all the Biblical sites and there were several highlights for me: being baptised in the River Jordan (total immersion), swimming in the Sea of Galilee, seeing a vision of three holy figures with halos over the leader's head while he was guiding a meditation on top of the Mount of Beatitudes. This was probably the event that made the most lasting impression. We were overlooking the Sea of Galilee, which was shimmering in the sunshine. The vision probably lasted for about thirty seconds and left me with the distinct feeling that 'all would be well, come what may'. I loved seeing the Chagall stained glass windows depicting the sons of Jacob in the University Chapel in Jerusalem. We also visited a site where the Essenes (an ascetic Jewish sect) had lived in Palestine 100 BC–100 AD. Several

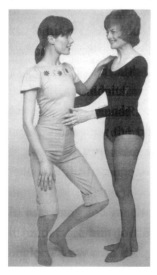

members of our group were convinced they had lived in those times and were scrambling around in the gravel looking for where they might have been buried in that life!

After the TV experience other possibilities for further programmes arose, but never materialised. It did, however, lead to radio work and more collaboration with journalists. One exciting prospect was teaching exercises on a Mediterranean cruise, but sadly it was cancelled because it coincided with difficult times in the economy so there were insufficient bookings.

Although I loved meeting such personalities as John Mills, also Rock Hudson and Paul Newman, both of whom stayed in the hotel while filming, Bob Hope, Vidal Sassoon, at least one prime minister and several politicians of the period, I realised I needed to find more creative satisfaction as apart from enjoying the social interaction at the hotel my work was mainly administrative. I had lived on a permanent adrenaline high throughout the TV series and have never felt so alive before or since, but was well aware of the inherent dangers in expecting the high to continue as the norm.

Meantime, I was contacted by the Head of the Beauty Therapy department at the London College of Fashion who asked me to teach exercise therapy and nutrition to the students. I was able to fit this in during my free time in the afternoons and found it stimulating to teach young girls (mothers of the future) how to become fit and then do the same for their clients. I asked to see the syllabus, but was told there wasn't one, which I thought odd so immediately set out to formulate one. The information must have been 'given' to me because come years later when challenged by an outside examiner (a previous teacher with an axe to grind) I produced my syllabus which was precisely as it should have been.

The syllabus was built on a foundation of anatomy and physiology and the course covered such subject areas as: the qualities and techniques required by a good teacher, the mechanics of movement, components of fitness, how to assess clients' fitness levels and devise suitable graded exercise programmes to suit individual needs. In addition, I taught the principles of nutrition and how to provide healthy eating plans to produce a predictable weight gain or loss or to maintain a given weight according to need. I have modified the routines I taught students and clients to demonstrate that, given sufficient determination, a satisfying result can be achieved by building a simple exercise routine into a busy working day. For those who find it difficult to establish the habit, the Seven-day plan and Daily Fitness Timetable in the following chapters have been designed to help readers take the first steps to a healthier lifestyle.

A balanced exercise routine

If you are having medical treatment, please check the suitability of an exercise programme with your doctor because there are certain conditions that make exercise inadvisable and others where a doctor's approval is necessary. Among them are pregnancy, extreme tiredness or general debility, high or low blood pressure, heart trouble, arteriosclerosis, high temperature, inflammation of the joints from a recent injury, rheumatoid or osteoarthritis, cartilage trouble in the knees, recent operation, recent childbirth, bronchitis, asthma or diabetes.

To achieve the best results, you will need to spend at least three, and for the quickest results, five or six 20–30 minute sessions per week exercising. Gradually this will:
* increase the efficiency of heart and lungs;
* lose you approximately 225 g–450 g per week through increased activity;
* improve flexibility, muscle tone/strength and shape;
* improve co-ordination and balance.

Some of the immediate benefits are:
* easier and quicker everyday movements, giving you more time to do other things;
* improved circulation, which will increase vitality and alertness and help regulate the appetite so that a poor one is stimulated and an excessive one will become more controlled;
* fewer aches and pains as postural awareness increases;
* more refreshing sleep.

Looseners
Purpose: To release excess stiffness and tension, and create warmth. By

using gravity and momentum they encourage normal relaxation after effort, which tense muscles have 'forgotten' to do. *Breathe* rhythmically and gently.

Gentle body stretch

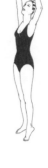

Method: Stand erect and raise the arms overhead. Reach up with the right arm while lifting the left heel, then with the left arm while lifting the right heel.

Repetitions: 3 each side.

Alternate arm circling

Method: Stand erect, feet a few inches apart and parallel. Alternately describe a large circle with each arm - forwards, up, back and down without twisting the trunk.

Repetitions: 6 each arm.

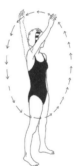

Shoulder straightener

Purpose: To stretch chest and firm upper back muscles; will correct a tendency to round shoulders and encourage deeper breathing.

Method: Stand erect, feet a few inches apart and parallel, arms raised forwards to chest level, elbows bent, fingertips almost touching, palms downwards. Extend the shoulders and move the elbows behind the trunk as far as possible, rebound to the first position. Repeat the movement with straight elbows and palms facing forwards (one cycle). Don't allow the head to push forwards. *Breathe* rhythmically throughout.

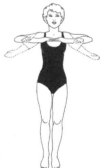

Repetitions: 6 cycles (by increasing the cycles from 15–20 this becomes a muscle firming exercise in which case place it before side bends).

Gentle jog

Method: Stand, shoulders relaxed, arms hanging loosely with elbows slightly bent, alternately lift each heel (keeping the ball of the foot and toes on the floor).

Repetitions: 5 times with each foot. Then gently lift each foot completely and continue with a gentle jog 10 times with each foot.

Trunk twists

Method: Stand erect, feet hip width apart and parallel; raise arms forwards to shoulder level. Twist 3 times to the right with a rebound in-between, each time aiming to twist a little further. Turn to face forwards and repeat to the left side (one cycle). It is important to move from the pelvis so that the arms, head and neck automatically follow in one smooth movement without jerking the head. Allow the leading arm to swing as far round as is comfortable.

Trunk side stretch

Method: Stand erect, feet approximately 18–24 in. apart and parallel, arms raised sideways to shoulder level. Turn left palm upwards, raise arm and allow it to relax over the head. Bend to the right side so that the right hand slides down towards the back of the outside of the thigh. Instead of actually pushing the right hand, when you feel the muscles stretching on the left side, consciously let go rather than resisting the pull. This way you will gradually move further without straining. Take your time, then straighten and repeat to the left side. Don't allow the trunk to bend forward.

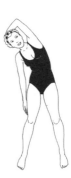

Breathe out as you bend sideways; pause while breathing in, make any necessary adjustments continuing the movement on the next out-breath and so on. Straighten up on an in-breath.

Repetitions: 3 each side.

Breathe in while raising arms, out while twisting to the sides and in when returning to the starting position.

Repetitions: 3 cycles.

Forward and backward leg swings

Method: Stand with the left hand resting lightly on a mantelpiece, shelf or similar support between shoulder and waist level. Swing the right leg forwards and backwards, straightening the knee gently on the forward swing and bending it gently on the backward swing. Turn around and repeat with the left leg.

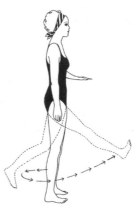

Repetitions: 6 times right leg, then 6 times left leg.

Note: On a cold day you may prefer to do the circulo-respiratory exercises next, otherwise continue with the firming and strengthening section that follows.

Trunk bend and straighten

Purpose: To increase flexibility in the lower back, the shoulders and the area behind the knees.

Method: Stand erect, feet 18–24 in. apart and parallel. Draw abdominal muscles in gently, raise arms sideways to shoulder level. Then bend forwards from the hips in a gentle bouncing motion, keeping the head and neck bent backwards and the spine straight. Hold the position for a few seconds, then relax the head, back, arms and knees and try to touch the floor first in front of the legs, then between the legs and lastly behind the legs. Straighten up, one vertebra at a time, starting from the

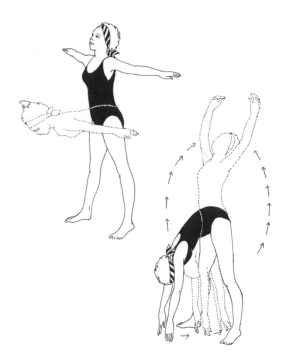

base of the spine, again with the abdominal muscles drawn in, bend backwards a little, bending the knees to help balance, and circle the arms up, back and down. Keep the knees relaxed on the forward bend if you are aware of the tension.

Breathe in while getting into position, out on the forward bend and in and out while straightening up and circling the arms.

Repetitions: 3.

Neck exercises

Purpose: To increase flexibility in the neck joints and release tension in the muscles so that they become evenly toned.

Forward and backward neck bends

Method: Sit comfortably erect either in a chair or on the floor, cross-legged, or kneel and sit on the heels. With the chin at right angles to neck, consciously drop the shoulders and rest hands in the lap. Lift the neck upwards, pull the chin inwards towards the neck and push the shoulders towards the floor, while very slowly bending the chin on to the chest.

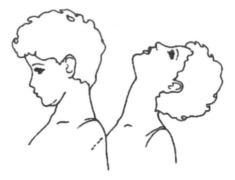

Try to bend the head only rather than the neck. If you don't feel the muscles stretching at the point where the head joins the neck, you are not doing the exercise properly. Release the stretch, straighten up and slowly bend the head back until it touches the back of the shoulders. Open the mouth wide, then close it, slowly raising the lower jaw as high as possible, then return to the starting position.

Neck twists

Method: Slowly turn the head and neck to the right, then to the left without tensing the shoulders.

Neck side bends

Method: Still facing forwards, slowly bend the head and neck towards the right shoulder without raising it. Then push the left shoulder towards the floor to increase the stretch. Straighten up and repeat to the left side. Notice whether the muscles feel tighter on one side than the other. If so, stretch the tighter side more times.

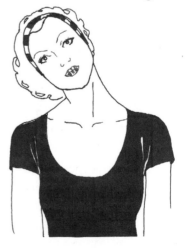

Neck circles

Method: Lift the neck upwards, pull the chin inwards and push the shoulders down, then bend the chin slowly to the chest, keeping the neck as erect as possible. Turn to the right, then bend the head back and complete the circle by turning to the left and touching the chest with the chin (one cycle). Repeat, turning first to the left.

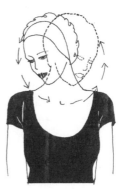

Breathe rhythmically throughout. If possible, breathe out when moving into a position – that is, forwards or backwards, twisting or bending to the side – and in when returning to the starting position.

Repetitions: average 3 and 1 to 3 cycles of the circles.

Muscle toning, firming and stretching

Wall press-ups

Purpose: To firm the chest and the back of upper arm muscles.

Method: Stand facing a wall, feet comfortably apart, and a few feet from the wall. Lean forwards, raising heels and place palms on the wall, fingertips pointing inwards, shoulder width apart. Trunk and legs should form a straight line, so draw abdominal muscles gently

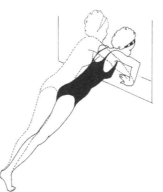

in and tuck buttocks under. Allow elbows to bend as much as possible, then push the hands both against the wall and also towards each other (it is the effort that counts – the hands don't actually need to move), then straighten up.

Note: If the heels are kept on the floor throughout, this will stretch tight calf muscles and Achilles tendons.

Breathe in as you move forwards and out while straightening up.

Repetitions: 8 to 10, gradually increasing to 20.

If, or when you can manage this easily, try the same movement resting hands on a mantelpiece or window ledge, progressing to a chest, table or chair height. Most men will be able to start at table height or below.

Side bends

Purpose: To lengthen and firm the waistline.

Method: Stand with feet 18–24 in. apart and parallel, right hand on ear, elbow bent in line with trunk and held well back. Bend to the left and slide left hand down outer thigh. Then swing over to the right side, aiming to place the right elbow on the right hip if possible. Be careful not to bend the trunk or head forwards, or to fling the head and neck from side to side; keep them still.

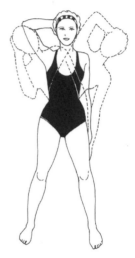

Breathe rhythmically throughout.

Repetitions: 10 with right hand on right ear, 10 with left hand on left ear, gradually increasing to 20 each side.

Alternatives: • If, in spite of keeping the head still, you feel dizzy for no medical reason, slow movement down and try the exercise either with arms at side or sit astride a chair or stool.

• If you tend to bend forwards or twist the trunk, stand with your back to the wall and keep your head, shoulders, arms, and buttocks in contact with the wall.

Knee extensions

Purpose: To firm and strengthen the front of thigh muscles and tendons attached to the knee joint.

Method: Sit erect on a hard-surfaced chair with a seat as deep as the length of the thighs so that the knee joint fits over the edge, or sit on a strong, high kitchen-type table so that the feet don't touch the floor. Place hands on either side of the chair seat (or if on a table over the front edge). Bend the knees as much as possible, then straighten them strongly, turn toes upwards so that there is a

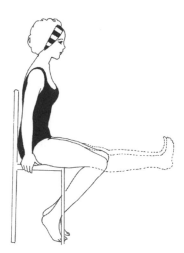

right angle between the foot and calf. Hold for a second and return to the starting position.

Breathe in to prepare, out on the lift, and in as the legs are lowered.

Repetitions: 8–10 according to ability, gradually increasing to 20, or 10 with a pause, then another 10.

Alternatives: • Same movement, but raise each leg alternately.
• Same movement, but work with one leg at a time, that is, 8–10 repetitions with one leg followed by 8–10 repetitions with the other leg.

Head, neck and upper trunk lifts from face downwards (prone) lying

Purpose: To firm back muscles.

Method: Lie face downwards on the floor and place arms on back. If necessary for comfort, place a folded towel or flat cushion under the pelvis. Lift head, and as much of trunk as possible, then return to the floor. Press your feet down or place them under a support (a low bed or chest, for example) to concentrate on lifting the trunk.

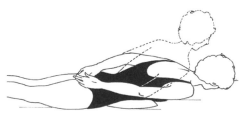

Note: You could do this exercise in pairs with your partner holding your feet down.

> *Breathe* in to prepare, out to lift, and in to return to the floor.

Repetitions: 5, gradually increasing to 10.

Half sit-ups

Purpose: To firm the abdominal area. Suitable for all ages and conditions, except a recent slipped disc in the neck.

Method: Lie on the back, soles of the feet on the floor, knees bent to form an approximate right angle (crook lying), palms resting on the front of the thighs. Tuck chin against the chest, draw in the abdominal muscles, then slide hands towards knees and lift the head, neck and, if possible, the shoulders. With continued practice, the shoulder-blades will lift off the floor, but don't heave or strain to do this. Hold the position for three seconds, then slowly return to the floor, vertebra by vertebra. If you feel particular discomfort in the neck, cradle it in a towel. With practice you will be able to hold the position for 5 seconds.

Breathe in to prepare, out as you lift up, in and out as you return to the floor and relax.

Repetitions: 5, gradually increasing to 10 and eventually to 20.

Leg lifts from face downwards lying

Purpose: To firm the buttocks.

Method: Lie face downwards, arms at the sides. (If the position causes discomfort in the lower back, place a folded towel or flat

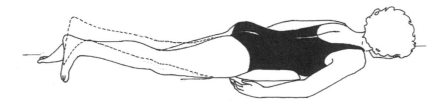

cushion under the pelvis to prevent an excessive hollow in the lumbar spine). Press the base of the pelvis downwards, clench right buttock, twist the leg outwards from the hip joint and lift *straight* up (not sideways) as high as possible. Hold for three seconds and lower to the floor. Now lift the left leg in the same manner (one cycle).

Note: Keep the knee well-braced when lifting the leg and keep the pelvis in contact with the floor.

Breathe in to prepare, out to lift and hold, in to lower.

Repetitions: 8 cycles, increasing to 15.

Hip rolls

Purpose: To increase pelvic flexibility, firm the waist and, to a lesser extent, create friction on the buttocks and outer thighs, thereby increasing circulation, hopefully removing waste products and helping the breakdown of fatty deposits.

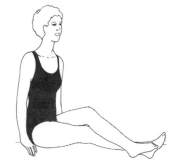

Method: Sit on the floor with legs straight, palms on the floor by the outer side of the upper thighs (not behind buttocks). Cross the left leg over the right just above the ankle. Then, keeping the left knee slightly bent, push off with the left hand and twist the pelvis to the right so that the left knee touches the floor, then push off with the right hand and twist the pelvis to the left so that the left knee again touches the floor. Repeat 10 times, then cross the right leg over the left and twist first to the left and then to the right 10 times. In order to control the movement, it is important to keep the feet in contact with each other, and to sit well forwards on the 'buttock bones'. There is then more body

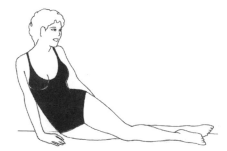

159

weight behind the movement to cause friction on the outer thighs and buttocks. Don't allow the hands to stray behind the buttocks.

Breathe rhythmically.

Repetitions: 10 in each leg position, gradually increasing to 20.

Upper leg lifts from side lying

Purpose: To firm outer hips and thighs.

Method: Lie on the left side, left arm extended along the floor beyond

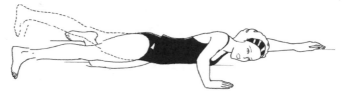

the head in line with the trunk and legs. Rest the head on the left shoulder and place the right hand on the floor at waist level. Twist the right leg inwards from the hip and place the foot at right angles to the calf. Toes should be on the floor and heel pointing diagonally upwards. Bend the left knee to form a right angle between lower leg and thigh. The left arm, head, trunk, left thigh and right leg should all be in a straight line. Without using downward pressure with the right hand or foot, lift the right leg up, concentrating the effort on the area from the outside of the knee to the hip joint. Hold the contraction for three seconds, then lower the leg to the floor; repeat eight to ten times. Repeat with the left leg.

Breathe in to prepare, out to lift and hold, in to return to the starting position.

Repetitions: 8–10, gradually increasing to 20.

Note: A common fault is to let the top hip roll backwards and then lift the leg forwards and up instead of sideways. The leg will lift higher, but it works the muscles in the lower abdomen and front of thighs instead of those at the side.

Under leg lifts from side lying

Purpose: To firm the inner thighs.

Method: Lie on the right side with the right arm extended along the floor beyond the head, the head resting on the shoulder, trunk and legs in a straight line. Place the left hand on the floor at waist level. Flex the left hip and place the leg from the knee downwards on the floor in front of the right leg. Keep the right foot at a right angle with the leg, brace the knee and lift the leg as high as possible, then hold for 3 seconds and lower to the floor. Repeat 8 to 9 times, according to ability. Repeat with the left leg. Take care not to tense the neck and shoulder muscles or push the supporting hand against the floor to 'help' lift the leg.

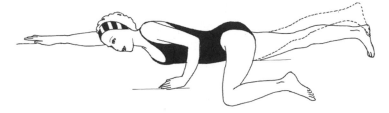

    Breathe in to prepare, out to lift and hold, in to lower.

Repetitions: 8 to ten, gradually increasing to 20.

Spinal rock

Purpose: To release any tension in the lower back.

Method: Lie on the back with feet on the floor and knees bent. Grasp the knees, lift the feet, head and neck and

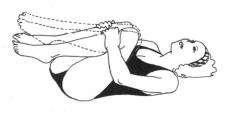

rock gently forwards and backwards so that the spine is gently massaged against the floor. Leave the head down if raising it makes the neck ache.

    Breathe rhythmically.

Repetitions: 5 approximately.

Circulo-respiratory efficiency

Time: Aim for 5 minutes or more.

Running on the spot

Purpose: Apart from the aerobic benefits, it strengthens ankle and
foot muscles, tones and shapes
the calf and thigh muscles.

Method: Stand erect, feet a few inches
apart and parallel, shoulders
relaxed and elbows bent. Start
by simply raising alternate
heels several times, then
continue by raising the feet

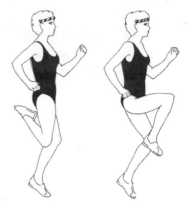

completely, just an inch or two, taking care to land gently (balls
of the feet followed by heels). Continue, this time raising the
knees as high as possible. Follow with more gentle movements,
then build up again, trying to kick the buttocks with the heels.
Finish with more gentle movements.

Breathe rhythmically throughout.

Repetitions: Start by lifting heels only 10 times – that is, 5 right heel, 5 left
heel.

- Gently with the whole foot 10 times
- Lifting the knees high 10 times
- Gently with the whole foot 10 times
- Kicking the buttocks 10 times
- Gently with the whole foot 10 times

Star jumps

Purpose: Similar to running on the spot. Also increases flexibility in the
shoulder area.

Method: Spring feet about 24 inches apart (lower the whole foot) and
clap hands together over head. Then spring back to the starting
position (count as one).

Breathe rhythmically.

Repetitions: 15, increasing to 25. Then repeat entire sequence, the running on the spot followed by star jumps several times for 1 to 3 minutes, as long as no discomfort is felt. Gradually increase speed and time for 5 minutes or more, aiming to maintain a pulse rate of 120 for 3 minutes. A simple guideline is to attain a degree of breathlessness that still enables you to talk easily or hum a tune.

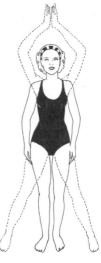

Warming-down stretches

Time taken: Aim for 3–10 minutes.

Purpose: To help speed the return of venous blood to the heart, also the removal of lactic acids produced by the working muscles.

Bicycling in the air

Purpose: In addition to the above, tones front of thigh and calf muscles; increases flexibility in the knees and ankles.

Method: Take up the crook-lying position. Keeping the arms straight, place them palms downwards under the back for support. Lift the feet and draw knees close to the chest. Straighten and bend each knee alternately as you 'pedal' in a vertical direction (one cycle). At the same time, 'square' and then 'point' each foot.

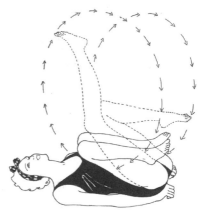

Breathe rhythmically throughout.

Repetitions: 10 cycles.

Gentle body stretch

Purpose: To release any tension in the shoulders, trunk and the area behind the knees.

Method: Lie on the back with the arms resting on the floor beyond the head. Push the right arm and left foot or right arm and right foot for a slightly different stretch (with foot square to the leg) away from the trunk. Stop pushing and allow the muscles to relax naturally – the elbows will bend slightly and the feet will flop sideways. Repeat on the other side.

Breathe out while pushing and in while relaxing.

Repetitions: 3 each side.

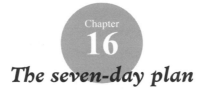

The seven-day plan

A daily fitness guide for the busy person

If I've stimulated readers to put my methods into practice, this seven-day plan has been devised to help you get started.

Since most of us start a new project at the beginning of the week, I am assuming Day 1 to be a Monday. Once you have established the habit, you will find a wider choice of exercise and nutritional advice in other relevant sections throughout the book.

Day 1
Thought for the day: *The three essentials for health and vitality are: think well, eat well, move well. – Mary Perigoe*

Tip: Record your measurements, weight, postural assessment and realistic aims in a form you find comfortable and easy to reference.

Exercise programme:

5 Minute stretches
Tip: It is a good idea to do them a second time during the day i.e. when you feel you need a break
1. Gentle body stretch, 3 each side
2. Alternate arm circling, 6 per arm
3. Trunk twists, 3 cycles
4. Trunk side stretch, 3 each side
5. Forward & backward leg swings, 6 per leg
6. Neck exercises, 3 cycles for each exercise

From tomorrow onwards, try doing the stretches before breakfast and leave the others for later if this is more convenient.

5 Minute muscle toning and strengthening

For real beginners there are just two exercises today and others are added during the week. If you're in better shape start with the Day 5 programme for a more thorough workout.

1. Wall/Windowsill press-ups, 8–10
2. Half sit-ups, 5
3. Gentle body stretch, 3 each side (from standing or lying positions)

Daily balanced diet

Adjust the food amounts proportionally to suit your individual calorie needs. Minimum daily requirements for an active person are approximately 1250–1500 calories.

- 170 g–227 g protein rich foods
- 397 g–454 g salad and vegetables
- 397 g–454 g fresh fruit
- 28 g–29 g butter or oil
- 57 g–113 g wholegrain foods i.e. bread, crispbread, rice and cereals
- 250 ml semi-skimmed milk or equivalent yogurt
- 1.5 L–2 L of water/juices from fruits, vegetables, herbal teas (excluding caffeinated drinks)

Tip: Try to unwind with a quiet leisure activity for at least an hour before bedtime. Practise gentle, even breathing as a preparation for sleep and whenever you feel stressed during the day.

Day 2

Thought for the day: *Time is the most valuable thing a man can spend. – Theophrastius*

Exercise programme:

5 Minute stretches

1. Gentle body stretch, 3 each side
2. Alternate arm circling, 6 per arm
3. Trunk twists, 3 cycles
4. Trunk side stretch, 3 each side

5. Forward & backward leg swings, 6 per leg
6. Neck exercises, 3 cycles for each exercise

8 Minute muscle toning and strengthening
1. Wall/Windowsill press-ups, 8–10
2. Half sit-ups, 5
3. Leg lifts, 8 cycles lying face down
4. Knee extensions, 8–10 per leg
5. Gentle body stretch, 3 each side (from standing or lying positions)

During the day take a brisk walk, holding yourself tall and breathing deeply (30 minutes or 2 x 15 minutes). Try for a 100–120 paces per minute.

Tip: Check your posture at regular intervals and practise the relevant posture exercises.

Daily balanced diet
Adjust the food amounts proportionally to suit your individual calorie needs. Minimum daily requirements for an active person are approximately 1250–1500 calories.
- 170 g–227 g protein rich foods
- 397 g–454 g salad and vegetables
- 397 g–454 g fresh fruit
- 28 g–29 g butter or oil
- 57 g–113 g wholegrain foods i.e. bread, crispbread, rice and cereals
- 250 ml semi-skimmed milk or equivalent yogurt
- 1.5 L–2 L of water/juices from fruits, vegetables, herbal teas (excluding caffeinated drinks)

Day 3
Thought for the day: *You can not help men permanently by doing for them what they could do for themselves. – Abraham Lincoln*

Exercise programme:
5 Minute stretches
1. Gentle body stretch, 3 each side

2. Alternate arm circling, 6 per arm
3. Trunk twists, 3 cycles
4. Trunk side stretch, 3 each side
5. Forward & backward leg swings, 6 per leg
6. Neck exercises, 3 cycles for each exercise

10 Minute muscle toning and strengthening
1. Wall/Windowsill press-ups, 8–10
2. Side bends, 5 per side
3. Half sit-ups, 5
4. Knee extensions, 8–10 per leg
5. Leg lifts, 8 cycles lying face down
6. Upper leg lifts from side lying, 8–10 (hold each lift for 3 seconds)
7. Gentle body stretch, 3 each side (from standing or lying positions)

Include a 30 minute brisk walk during the day.

Daily balanced diet
Adjust the food amounts proportionally to suit your individual calorie needs. Minimum daily requirements for an active person are approximately 1250–1500 calories.
- 170 g–227 g protein rich foods
- 397 g–454 g salad and vegetables
- 397 g–454 g fresh fruit
- 28 g–29 g butter or oil
- 57 g–113 g wholegrain foods i.e. bread, crispbread, rice and cereals
- 250 ml semi-skimmed milk or equivalent yogurt
- 1.5 L–2 L of water/juices from fruits, vegetables, herbal teas (excluding caffeinated drinks)

Day 4
Thought for the day: *Achievement lags behind desire in any person who is growing. – Robert Browning*

Exercise programme:

5 Minute stretches
1. Gentle body stretch, 3 each side
2. Alternate arm circling, 6 per arm
3. Trunk twists, 3 cycles
4. Trunk side stretch, 3 each side
5. Forward & backward leg swings, 6 per leg
6. Neck exercises, 3 cycles for each exercise

10 Minute muscle toning and strengthening
1. Wall/Windowsill press-ups, 8–10
2. Side bends, 10 per side
3. Half sit-ups, 5
4. Knee extensions, 8–10 per leg
5. Leg lifts, 8 cycles lying face down
6. Upper leg lifts from side lying, 8–10 (hold each lift for 3 seconds)
7. Under leg lifts from side lying, 8–10 (hold each lift for 3 seconds)
8. Gentle body stretch, 3 each side (from standing or lying positions)

Include a 30 minute brisk walk during the day. Try alternating 50 fast walking steps with 50 easy jogging steps.

Tip: Make use of extra opportunities to stretch and exercise while doing housework; use stairs instead of lifts; walk up an escalator and so on.

Daily balanced diet
Adjust the food amounts proportionally to suit your individual calorie needs. Minimum daily requirements for an active person are approximately 1250–1500 calories.
- 170 g–227 g protein rich foods
- 397 g–454 g salad and vegetables
- 397 g–454 g fresh fruit
- 28 g–29 g butter or oil
- 57 g–113 g wholegrain foods i.e. bread, crispbread, rice and cereals
- 250 ml semi-skimmed milk or equivalent yogurt

- 1.5 L–2 L of water/juices from fruits, vegetables, herbal teas (excluding caffeinated drinks)

Day 5
Thought for the day: *Tomorrow's strength is very largely the heritage of today's patient striving. – Keble*

Exercise programme:

5 Minute stretches
1. Gentle body stretch, 3 each side
2. Alternate arm circling, 6 per arm
3. Trunk twists, 3 cycles
4. Trunk side stretch, 3 each side
5. Forward & backward leg swings, 6 per leg
6. Neck exercises, 3 cycles for each exercise

10 Minute muscle toning and strengthening
1. Wall/Windowsill press-ups, 8–10
2. Side bends, 10 per side
3. Half sit-ups, 5
4. Knee extensions, 8–10 per leg
5. Head, neck and upper trunk lifts from face downwards lying, 5–7
6. Leg Lifts, 8 cycles lying face down
7. Upper leg lifts from side lying, 8–10 (hold each lift for 3 seconds)
8. Under leg lifts from side lying, 8–10 (hold each lift for 3 seconds)
9. Gentle body stretch, 3 each side (from standing or lying positions)

Take a brisk walk/jog alternating between them every 50 paces. Include at least 1–3 minutes of aerobics: Running on the spot, alternating with star jumps or repeat the combined brisk walk and jog.

Tip: Plan some joint sporting or other physical activities with the family such as tennis, swimming, games, walking or gardening – watch your posture

*and alternate jobs to prevent backache etc. Adjust your weekend shopping
list along healthier lines.*

Day 6

Thought for the day: *Think of your body as the temple in which your soul
lives and care for it accordingly. – Mary Perigoe*

Exercise programme:

5 Minute stretches
1. Gentle body stretch, 3 each side
2. Alternate arm circling, 6 per arm
3. Trunk twists, 3 cycles
4. Trunk side stretch, 3 each side
5. Forward & backward leg swings, 6 per leg
6. Neck exercises, 3 cycles for each exercise

Also, at some time during the day take a brisk walk, alternating to a gentle
jog every 50 paces with a friend or with the family.

Watch your posture when shopping and make necessary adjustments.

10 Minute muscle toning and strengthening
1. Wall/Windowsill press-ups, 8–10
2. Side bends, 10 per side
3. Half sit-ups, 5
4, Knee extensions, 8–10 per leg
5. Head, neck and upper trunk lifts from face downwards lying, 5–7
6. Leg lifts, 8 cycles lying face down
7. Upper leg lifts from side lying, 8–10 (hold each lift for 3 seconds)
8. Under leg lifts from side lying, 8–10 (hold each lift for 3 seconds)
9. Gentle body stretch, 3 each side (from standing or lying positions)

*Tip: Remain as close as possible to your eating programme without feeling
deprived. Adjust your recipes to include less fats and sugar and more fruits
and vegetables, but not so drastically that the family protests.*

Day 7

Thought for the day: *The reward for a thing well done is to have done it.*
– R. W. Emerson

Exercise programme:

5 Minute stretches
1. Gentle body stretch, 3 each side
2. Alternate arm circling, 6 per arm
3. Trunk twists, 3 cycles
4. Trunk side stretch, 3 each side
5. Forward & backward leg swings, 6 per leg
6. Neck exercises, 3 cycles for each exercise

Sometime during the day take a brisk walk, alternating to a gentle jog every 50 paces.

10 Minute muscle toning and strengthening
1. Wall/Windowsill press-ups, 8–10
2. Side bends, 10 per side
3. Half sit-ups, 5
4. Knee extensions, 8–10 per leg
5. Head, neck and upper trunk lifts from face downwards lying, 5–7
6. Leg lifts, 8 cycles lying face down
7. Upper leg lifts from side lying, 8–10 (hold each lift for 3 seconds)
8. Under leg lifts from side lying, 8–10 (hold each lift for 3 seconds)
9. Gentle body stretch, 3 each side (from standing or lying positions)

Tip: Review the week's progress noting both problems and improvements such as increased energy, increased elimination and increased joint flexibility. Study the text for further suggestions to follow such as balancing your colour energies through your choice of foods.

Variations of the seven-day plan

If you've found this plan useful, continue to use it as a daily reminder, gradually increase the repetitions of the toning/strengthening exercises and, when appropriate, include the progressions and other exercises found in the exercise plan.

During a period of stress, overwork, or while on holiday, you may give up the routine. At the very least, follow a thought tip, an exercise tip and a food tip. Choose from the following selection, then add some ideas of your own or highlight phrases in the text appropriate for your needs. As soon as possible, ease back to a more effective routine.

Seven examples of daily tips

Thought tip

No one can make you feel inferior without your own consent. – Eleanor Roosevelt

Exercise tip

Walk tall and hold your ears immediately above your shoulders. Keep your shoulders relaxed at all times.

Food tip

Chew each mouthful of food thoroughly to aid digestion and enjoy the full flavour.

Thought tip

Man's reach must exceed his grasp, or what's a heaven for? – Robert Browning

Exercise tip

Back slide: Stand with the back of your head and entire back from shoulders downwards against a wall, feet about 12 inches in front and comfortably apart. Slide your spine down and up 10 times bending and straightening the knees alternately (pointed over the feet), at the same time lifting and lowering the heels.

Food tip

Include at least two pieces of ripe, fresh fruit in your daily diet.

Thought tip

We must always change, review, rejuvenate ourselves otherwise we harden. – Goethe

Exercise tip

Walk briskly in the fresh air for at least 30 minutes, breathing regularly.

Food tip

Cut down your salt intake and use more fresh or dried herbs for flavouring.

Thought tip

Trust but verify. – Ronald Reagan

Exercise tip

To keep the neck flexible, turn the head slowly and comfortably from side to side 3 – 6 times each way.

Food tip

Drink at least 4 glasses of water per day, mostly between meals and not more than one glass with a meal so as not to delay digestion.

Thought tip

Those who bring sunshine into the lives of others cannot keep it from themselves. – J. M. Barrie

Exercise tip

Shoulder straightener: Stand feet a few inches apart and parallel. Raise arms forward to chest level, with elbows bent. Swing elbows behind body as far as possible and rebound to starting position, repeat the movement with straight elbows and palms facing forward 10 times.

Food tip

Eat some fresh salad material or raw vegetables such as watercress and carrots each day.

Thought tip

Our glory is not in never falling but in rising each time we fall. – Confucius

Exercise tip

During your daily walk, clench the buttocks strongly for at least 50 consecutive steps, to firm the buttocks.

Food tip

Avoid salted nuts and crisps as appetisers. Substitute sticks of celery, cucumber, carrots, peppers, or unsalted nuts and raisins in limited quantities.

Thought tip

No man is free who cannot command himself. – Pythagoras

Exercise tip

To help prevent or relieve eye-strain, rest the eyes periodically by sitting with elbows bent and placed on a cushion; cover the eyes lightly with the palms and relax for 10 minutes.

Food tip

Choose your food portions in the following descending order: vegetables, fruit, protein (fish, meat, eggs, cheese etc), carbohydrates (bread, rice, cereals etc), fats and oils (butter, olive and cold-pressed vegetable oils).

A daily fitness timetable

- On waking: Stretch gently several times and immediately recall any significant dreams that may contribute to the resolution of long-standing problems.

- Record any answers to current problems that come to mind on awakening.

- Contemplate your day ahead and adjust plans where necessary.

- Anticipate possible difficulties and consider how best to cope with them.

- On arising: Do some loosening exercises by an open window (such as gentle stretches, alternate arm circling and shoulder straightener). At the same time, breathe evenly and deeply. Sip a glass of water (hot or cold, with two tsp cider vinegar and one tsp honey or fresh juice if preferred).

- Follow your bath or shower with a vigorous rub-down, using a rough towel to remove dead cells and allow the pores to breathe freely.

- BREAKFAST is an important preparation for an efficient morning's work so if you're tempted to skip it, have a bowl of unsweetened muesli with milk or plain yoghurt and fresh fruit or make it a liquidised meal such as milk, banana and yoghurt.

- Walk part of the way to work or walk up an escalator or flights of stairs.

- During the working day take time to identify your nervous and muscular reactions to stressful situations. Adopt gentler and more positive attitudes, effortlessly balanced postures and slower more even breathing patterns.

- Take regular breaks, noting your energy highs and lows and learn to distinguish between the need for a rest, to quench your thirst, satisfy a real hunger or to change your activity.

- AT LUNCHTIME, make a wise choice of foods to maintain a high energy level through the working day and recognise that eating too little usually leads to non-stop eating during the evening.

- Note the time of day when your brain is less efficient and situations that make you nervously tense. Exercising then will revitalise the brain and calm the nerves. Otherwise, choose to exercise when your physical energies are relatively high. Exercising after work (before the evening meal) helps many office workers re-charge their batteries.

- Make time for hobbies or, at least, include a leisure activity every day, even if it's only browsing in a bookshop or art gallery, or admiring the beauties of nature.

- A walk before bedtime (walking the dog for instance) can relax the mind and prepare the body for sleep.

- Quietly unwind an hour before retiring to bed, review the day that has passed and make any necessary preparations for the next day.

- Delegate unsolved problems to your higher mind if you require guidance, or to your subconscious mind if you need to recall information from your memory, by making a simple verbal request for the help you need.

- Spend a few moments in quiet contemplation, breathing gently, listening to calming music, saying your prayers or making a positive affirmation such as: *I am a part of the universal mind and can attract like a magnet all the help I need.*

- Have a pen and paper beside the bed to record important last minute thoughts and answers to problems that may come to you on awakening. You may also find it useful to recall significant dreams which can shed light on unfinished business from your recent or distant past.

Keeping up the good work

After two to three months of regular exercise you will realise more than ever that the body is designed for movement and you will no longer avoid it like your unfit friends. You will be loath to let your body organs and systems become less efficient and will appreciate that tiredness and lethargy are more likely to be due to overweight or mental tension than physical activity.

As your everyday movements become faster and easier, maintaining your new found fitness should present no problems. Apart from a nutritionally and calorie balanced diet to maintain your ideal weight, you need to combine a regular energetic sport or two to three 20–30 minute exercise sessions per week, with some of the following every day:
- Move your major joints through their full range.
- Welcome every opportunity to stretch to top shelves, or while hanging out the washing.
- Bend the knees to open cupboards and drawers.
- Rub dry more briskly after a bath or shower.
- Squeeze out the flannel forcefully.
- Polish the furniture (with each hand).
- Scrub a floor (with each hand).
- Walk up stairs and escalators (down is only a third as good).
- Walk more briskly when carrying heavy bags or shopping (but make sure posture remains erect and the load is evenly distributed).
- Statically contract abdominal, buttock, pectoral and upper arm muscles.
- Stand at least 2 hours per day, not necessarily all at once, to strengthen bone structure, postural muscles and help blood pressure to adjust to changes in body positions.

Try to burn up approximately 300 calories with the types of activity listed in the table below and include energetic activities such as running for a bus, and so on.

Approximate calories burnt in physical exercise

	Calories
Walking up 20 flights of stairs (down uses only 1/3 as much)	50
Walking 1½ miles	100
Walking ¾ mile briskly (i.e. 100–120 paces per minute)	100
30 minutes brisk walk	200
Combination of 5 minutes running or skipping, and 10 minutes mobility and strengthening exercises	100

		Per minute
Standard walk (i.e. 3½–4 mph)		5–6
Brisk walk 4–4½ mph		5–6
Walking upstairs		6
Easy jog		10
Tennis, moderate effort		6
Ballroom dancing		4+
Square dancing (energetic)		10
Disco-type		10
Running	5½ mph	12
	7 mph	14.5
Skipping	70–80 jumps	15
Swimming, e.g		
breast stroke	2¼ mph	30.8
backstroke	2¼ mph	33.3

Note: If you give up exercising altogether you will gradually lose all the benefits you gained. The above figures apply to someone weighing 150 lb. For every 15 lb. over or under this weight add or deduct 10%.

Further tips for losing weight

- **Record good reactions** to your exercise and diet programmes.
- **Get sufficient** rest and deep, relaxed sleep.
- **Contemplate the extra pounds** you have lost or have still to lose in the form of canned foods, packets of butter or sugar or bags of potatoes.
- **Display a 'fat' photograph**; make it as hideous as possible.
- **Make up a list of the advantages** of being slim and disadvantages of being overweight.
- **Try on favourite 'slim'** clothes that no longer fit.
- **Refuse** to buy a larger size of clothes.
- **Decide whether the group therapy of slimming clubs**, the encouragement of a therapist or going it alone is most likely to help you.
- **When tired or tense**, instead of resorting to food, try locking yourself in the bathroom, as I have done, and unwind while you soak in the bath with some delicious oil or perfume sprinkled on the bath water. Alternatively, if you have the presence of mind to avoid going to the fridge, lie on your bed, or on the floor on your back with your calves and feet resting on an armchair with your thighs perpendicular to the floor. You could also sit down, play some soothing music and sip an unsweetened fruit juice. When tired, it is often impossible to distinguish between the need to eat, drink or rest. If you avoid shopping for food when you are particularly tired or tense, you will not be tempted to buy the wrong foods. Try some relaxing exercises; you can progress to the more energetic ones when sufficient energy is restored.
- **Plan some enjoyable activity to follow meals** – going for a long purposeful walk, for instance. If you don't enjoy walking for its own sake, choose a sport, dancing or a creative hobby. If you are staying at home, find something to do that uses the hands or is otherwise too absorbing for you to be able to think of food. To make it easier to switch from food, get up from the meal table and straight away clean the teeth.
- **Utilise everyday ways of burning more calories**; use stairs, running up if you can, instead of using lifts; walk more often and more briskly. Welcome active jobs about the house – stretch, clean and polish. Practise correct posture and automatically contract abdominal muscles as often as possible.

- **When entertaining**, plan the menu so that you appear to be eating normal quantities of suitable food. Then you will not draw attention to yourself. Don't deprive yourself too much otherwise you will be tempted to eat titbits later. Be strong-minded and eat legitimate 'bits' as part of your calorie-controlled diet and not as 'extras'.
- **Eating in restaurants** should present no problems. As a starter, choose something like melon or smoked salmon (but be sparing with the bread and butter) or a prawn cocktail with very little mayonnaise. If you cannot or don't wish to avoid wine, drink it very slowly so that your glass will not have to be refilled too often.

  For a main course, choose grilled or poached fish, chicken or lean meat with a salad or green vegetables, no potatoes of course.

  For a dessert, choose fresh fruit or fresh fruit salad with little or no cream or sugar. Have black coffee if you wish or coffee with very little cream. Either avoid petit fours or limit yourself to one and refuse liqueurs.
- **At a dinner party**, eat and drink slowly, avoiding sauces, cream, sugar and pastry wherever possible. At the same time, try not to draw attention to yourself. After indulgence, aim to eat very little the next day. A fruit and yogurt diet or a liquid-only diet until early supper are both good ideas.
- **If you have a teenage family**, avoid cooking separate meals. Instead, eat only the protein and vegetables and avoid pastries, potatoes other than those in their jackets occasionally; avoid sauces and plan a separate fruit and yogurt or stewed fruit dessert. Try to go easy on things like pie pastry and crumble, although some people spread 500 calories over both breakfast and lunch so that there is ample left for their evening meal.
- **If you have very young children** and cannot avoid nursery teas, try including a few legitimate 'healthy' titbits that your children will also enjoy. You could perhaps include some dainty open sandwiches and a few celery and carrot sticks and make this your one bread meal of the day.
- **If you are tempted to try a crash diet** for a short time, remember that apart from the odd day or if you have more than 7 lb. to lose overall, it is best that your protein foods should never fall below 6–8 oz/170–225 g a day. This will prevent your skin becoming loose or your losing the

strength from your muscles; it will also help cell renewal and therefore be less ageing. Always include a wide variety of salad or cooked vegetables to ensure sufficient vitamins and minerals, not less than ½ oz fat, 1 oz crispbread, wholegrain bread or cereal, and ¼ pt/140 ml of milk or the equivalent in yogurt. I also recommend a balanced vitamin and mineral pill from a health food shop.

- **Other aids that you might find useful** are biochemic tissue salts obtainable from health food shops. The Nat. Sulph. and Nat. Mur. combination will help remove the excess liquids; Cal. Phos. and Cal. Fluor. are particularly helpful if you have a great deal of weight to lose. Cal. Fluor. will help to avoid stretch marks and flabby muscles and Cal. Phos. will help prevent nutritional deficiency.
- **Overweight people who possibly have a slow metabolism** and suffer from liquid retention are often helped by a vitamin pill that includes vitamin B6, lecithin, and kelp.
- **Use nutritional boosters such as** kelp or wheat germ in casseroles and other cooked food to satisfy hidden hunger instead of useless foods such as sweets, chocolates, soft drinks, and some processed foods.
- **To avoid slimline eating becoming an extra expense**, try replacing expensive cuts of meat and fish with some of the following: brown rice, soya beans, lentils, whole barley, millet, sunflower seeds, sesame seeds, raw peanuts (unsalted), almonds, kidney, brain, heart and liver, all of which are cheaper than the organ meats, and are nutritionally superior to muscle meats.
- **Remove fat from meat** and remove skin (as the fat is under the skin) of chicken.
- **Use healthy calorie cutting alternatives:**
  - Substitute plain yogurt for cream. Low fat yogurt has had sugar added so is not necessarily a healthier alternative.
  - Use 'slimline' salad cream or cider vinegar or lemon juice.
  - Use herbs, Marmite, Barmene or Vecon (vegetable yeast extracts) for gravies usually made with fat and flour.
  - Substitute cottage or curd cheese for cream cheese; Cheshire, Edam or fat-reduced hard cheese for Cheddar.
  - Use skimmed or semi-skimmed instead of whole milk.

- Substitute wheat germ for uncooked muesli – the toasted oats variety is particularly condensed – weigh 30 g and you will see what I mean.
- Use tinned fish in brine instead of oil.
- Use tinned fruit in natural juices, or alternatively discard the syrup which will be high in sugar.
- **Prepare 'all in one' meals** either to eat at home or to put into a container to take to work. The following suggestions are suitable for one meal or as the basis for a one-day diet:
  - Mix together one 140 ml carton cottage cheese with 55 g chopped cooked beetroot, one teaspoon parsley and mint, chopped, and the juice of half a lemon (approximately 200 calories).
  - One 140 ml carton plain yogurt with one heaped tsp honey (approximately 120 calories); 5 fl oz yogurt with one medium-sized finely sliced banana (approximately 170 calories); 5 fl oz yogurt with one medium-sized peach, sliced with the skin left on and 1–2 shredded almonds (approximately 210 calories) or yogurt with 3 chopped walnuts and 1 oz raisins (approximately 250 calories).
  - Mix together 85 g shredded white cabbage, ½ grapefruit, pulp finely chopped, 2 tbsp yogurt, 1 tsp (level) paprika. Toss well together (approximately 70 calories), and serve with 85 g cold lamb (approximately 250 calories) or 85 g/3 oz cold roast chicken, without skin (160 calories).
  - Mix together one 140 ml/5 fl oz carton cottage cheese with six chopped walnuts, one stick celery finely chopped, and one medium-sized eating apple, cored and chopped but unpeeled (approximately 290 calories).
  - Mix together 85 g/3 oz chopped cold chicken (without skin) with 2 tbsp grated carrot, 85 g/3 oz finely shredded white cabbage, one tbsp low-calorie salad dressing, one stick celery, finely chopped, one medium-sized eating apple, cored and chopped but unpeeled, or 55 g/2 oz raisins 55 g/2 oz grapes (approximately 300 calories). If liked, use 3 oz tuna fish, drained of any oil, instead of the chicken.
  - Mix together 55 g/2 oz shredded white cabbage, one medium-sized carrot, finely grated, one small onion, peeled and chopped, one orange, peeled and the pulp finely chopped, 25 g/1 oz raisins, one tbsp each

of vegetable oil and cider vinegar. Toss well together. Sprinkle with 25 g/1 oz grated cheddar cheese (approximately 430 calories).

- One cucumber, half peeled and finely sliced, mixed with 3 medium-sized eating apples, cored and chopped but skins left on, 3 sticks celery, finely chopped, ½ small cauliflower, divided into small pieces, 3 medium-sized pears, peeled, cored and cut into small pieces, one small onion, peeled and chopped, 4 walnuts, chopped, one tsp chopped parsley. Dress with 1 tbsp lemon juice (approximately 490 calories). Suitable for two meals.

- Peel and remove some of the pith from 5 oranges and 5 grapefruit, cut the pulp into thin slices. Add 4 chopped walnuts, one tsp chopped parsley and one heaped tbsp honey. Pour over one tbsp lemon juice. Toss well together (approximately 515 calories). Suitable for two to three meals.

- Mix together 4 large bananas, sliced, 4 oranges, peeled and the pulp cut into slices, 3 tbsp finely grated carrot, 55 g/2 oz raisins. Toss well. Pour over 140 ml/5 fl oz carton plain yogurt mixed with 25 g/1 oz very finely chopped almonds (approximately 940 calories). Suitable for two to three meals.

• In cold weather, try slightly sweet salads; 1 tbsp grated carrot and a few sultanas sprinkled over shredded white cabbage with cider vinegar dressing, for instance.

'Near perfect' foods, (that supply a balance of essential nutrients) include: unpasteurised milk, or yogurt made with live culture; orange juice and yolk of egg, dates.

Tips to prevent nutritional loss

Vitamin A – not water-soluble but can be destroyed by preservatives in canned foods and by light and air (oxygen). Heat, when combined with air, also causes rapid oxidation and destruction. The same applies to pro-vitamin A (carotene), which is converted to vitamin A by the liver and is found in orange, yellow and dark green vegetables and fruit.

Vitamin B complex – among the most fragile group of nutrients along with vitamin C, B vitamins are lost in varying degrees by being dissolved in water. They are also destroyed by light, heat and alkaline substances, such as bicarbonate of soda (used as a colour preservative) and baking soda.

Vitamins B2 and nicotinic acid (niacin) – more stable in heat than the rest of the vitamin B complex.

Vitamin C – easily destroyed like the B-complex vitamins. Vitamin C can also be destroyed through oxidation, the process whereby oxygen is combined with other substances and produces toxic by-products (oxides). These can be neutralised by vitamin C, which is sacrificed in the process. Copper utensils have this effect and should be avoided. The vitamin C in green vegetables is destroyed by an enzyme if the leaves are allowed to wither or get crushed.

Vitamin D – lost in very high temperatures although it does not dissolve in water. The vitamin D produced by sunlight on the skin is often lost through air pollution.

Vitamin E – lost through heat, alkaline substances and light.

Vitamin K – lost in the freezing process.

Minerals – dissolve in water, so can be lost if the water in which food is boiled is thrown away. Overheating reduces the availability of calcium, for example in boiled milk and, to varying degrees, in the making of yogurt and cheese. Conversely, calcium in cereals may be more readily available when they are cooked.

Starch – in cereals and grains is made more digestible through cooking, although some vitamin B1 will be lost from these foods, depending on the degree of heat and the length of cooking time. The same applies to the starch in cooked flour preparations, bread and toast.

Protein – the value is reduced slightly during the canning process. Vitamins B1, B6, pantothenic acid, B12 and, to a lesser extent, B2 and niacin will be destroyed in cooked protein foods such as cheese, eggs, meat and poultry. Vitamin B1 and some minerals are leached into the water when boiling fish, but most of the vitamins A and D will be retained when cooking fatty fish such as herrings, sprats or salmon.

Fats and oils – and foods containing them such as seeds and nuts, lose their nutrients when exposed to heat and light and become rancid. Rancidity, not readily detected by taste, is an oxidation process and creates toxins in the body that damage healthy cells, a factor in the ageing process and disease. Rancid oils become cloudy and will throw up a white deposit when refrigerated. Store fats and oils away from light and heat and never re-use frying oils.

Extra precautions to minimise nutrient losses:
- If you grow your own produce, try to balance the mineral content of the soil naturally with compost. Avoid the use of insecticides and artificial fertilisers.
- Pick fruit and vegetables at their peak, immediately before use.
- Eat fruit and vegetables raw if possible, otherwise short-cook them.
- If you cannot grow your own, buy fresh, organically grown produce when possible (avoid those exposed to traffic fumes). Wash, dry and

wrap them (not with aluminium foil on account of possible long-term poisoning) after buying and store them in a cool, dark place, preferably in washable airtight containers. Cling film when in close contact with food is known to release plasticisers – potential carcinogens into its contents, particularly in the case of fatty foods such as cheese and meat.

- Buy frozen foods (usually prepared at peak freshness) in preference to withered or damaged produce.
- Scrub and scrape vegetables, though it is preferable to peel vegetables and fruit if they have been exposed to insecticides. A quick wash in water to which cider vinegar (approximately 1 dsp) has been added may help to remove the traces and will not affect the taste. Wash, but don't discard the outer green leaves of vegetables; they are rich in vitamins A and C. The thin parts of the leaves, incidentally, contain more iron than the ribbed parts.
- Cook potatoes in their skins. Dried potato and pre-cut chipped potatoes are treated with sulphite to preserve their colour. Vitamin C is retained but vitamin B1 is lost.
- When cooking vegetables, steam them or plunge them into very little boiling water and simmer with the lid on for the minimum time, and use any remaining liquid as stock. Vegetables that are pre-heated or kept hot for 30 minutes will lose all their vitamin C.
- Use very little salt in cooking. To avoid leaching of vitamins B and C and minerals, add it after draining the water rather than during cooking. Don't use bicarbonate of soda to preserve the colour of vegetables.
- Thaw frozen vegetables in boiling water. Thawing them slowly can destroy up to 50 per cent of the vitamin C. Pack frozen vegetables tightly; they lose fewer nutrients in storage.
- Prepare fruit and vegetable salads immediately before eating or cover with cling film and place in the fridge. Don't soak the fruit or vegetables, and cut them up as little as possible. A covering of cider vinegar or lemon juice will lessen plant enzyme activity and the effect of oxygen in destroying vitamins B and C.
- Buy fresh, unprocessed oils, fats, cheese, nuts and seeds, and avoid those exposed to heat or strong lighting on display. Add the contents of a vitamin E capsule to your cooking oils to preserve their freshness. Cover

and refrigerate fats or fatty foods immediately. Once cooked, avoid reheating them.

- Buy tuberculin-tested, unpasteurised milk when possible (sometimes available in country districts). Pasteurisation and sterilisation especially, incur losses of vitamins B and C. Never leave milk exposed to light and air; keep it in the fridge.
- Eat untoasted bread or cut thicker slices for toast since this cuts the loss of vitamin B1.
- Use glass cooking utensils with caution. They conduct heat slowly and help destroy vitamins B and C by exposure to light. Fruit juice, stored in clear glass bottles and left in the light, will lose its vitamin C. Unlined copper utensils, including knives which contain copper, will discolour and cause the loss of vitamin C.
- Avoid canned foods as much as possible; the high temperatures used in the process will destroy some vitamins. Never leave food in opened cans – metals such as lead and cadmium can leach from the seam when the contents are exposed to air.
- Avoid processed cake mixes that contain refined flour and sugar as well as artificial flavouring, colouring and preservatives.
- When buying crispbread, choose wholewheat or rye varieties and avoid those containing high levels of salt.
- When buying biscuits, remember quality is better than quantity. Develop a taste for those containing wholegrains, nuts and dried fruits. Avoid those containing a lot of sugar and salt.
- Read food labels carefully to ensure that you know exactly what each bottle, can and packet contains. Avoid those where additives come high up on the list.

Factors that affect food absorption

Eating a balanced diet is only half the story. Equal emphasis should be given to the state of the digestive tract and to the way food is handled once it is in the body. Poor absorption can mean that your body fails to utilise important nutrients, leading over time to chronic bad health.

Hasty eating and drinking

Milk and fruit juices should be sipped slowly. Bread, cereals and other carbohydrate and starch-containing foods, including fruits and vegetables, should be chewed to a pulp. If this is not done, the digestive juices in the mouth will be unable to break the foods down into usable nutrients.

Heavy physical work and activity

Because the process of digestion is slowed down during heavy physical work (blood is diverted away from the digestive tract to the muscles), it is strongly advised that you don't eat a main meal just before exercise.

Temperature

Iced food and drink lowers the temperature in the alimentary canal – normally 100 °F (37 °C) – and will therefore delay digestion.

Emotion

Don't eat or drink when you are worried, afraid, angry, over-heated, chilled or in pain. The digestive juices will not be secreted normally, and the hormones and other chemicals secreted during emotional crises will interfere with their functions. Relaxed pleasant feelings, on the other hand, actually aid digestion.

Food combining

Indigestion can result from eating foods that require different digestive enzymes at the same meal. Protein, for instance, requires hydrochloric acid in the stomach; starch requires the alkaline juices of the mouth and intestines. Try to take note if you frequently suffer from flatulence, stomach pains or feel bloated or sleepy after particular food combinations. These reactions are most likely to occur when you mix concentrated protein such as meat or fish with concentrated starch and sugar such as bread and pastry, as in meat pie or fruit pie with sugar. Hydrochloric acid is more concentrated in the bottom half of the stomach, so by eating the protein part first then the starch, the starch will be less likely to come into contact with the hydrochloric acid. Green vegetables and salads, being less concentrated, will combine with most other foods, as will fats as long as they are eaten in small amounts.

Very sweet fruits such as ripe bananas and dates combine with starch and sugar, but you may find that most fruit, especially citrus fruit, is best eaten on its own. It usually passes through the stomach in around 90 minutes and if eaten with other foods, this may be delayed and the food may be improperly digested.

Dried peas, beans and lentils can cause severe flatulence because they have a fairly even concentration of protein and starch. They are more easily digested when diluted in soups with other vegetables. Foods that are not properly digested will be decomposed by bacteria and form excess mucus. Bacterial breakdown may cause the stomach contents to putrefy and produce histamine, which causes an allergic reaction and destroys vitamin B1.

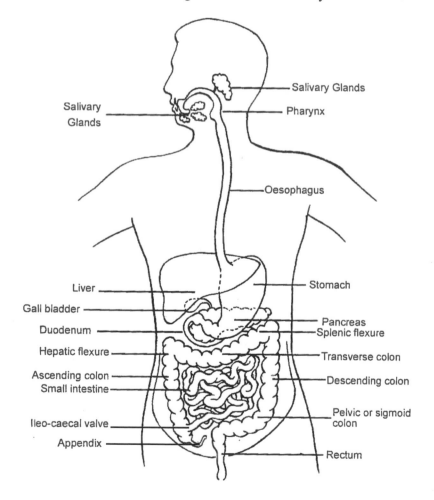

Mineral interactions

Eating foods plentiful in minerals does not necessarily mean that the body will absorb them all. Sodium, potassium and chlorine are absorbed easily, but calcium, magnesium and phosphorus are partly combined in complexes that are incompletely absorbed. Iron, copper, zinc, cobalt and manganese are also difficult to absorb in the form in which they enter the body. Phytic acid, for instance, found in wheat, oats and other cereals, is known to interfere with calcium, zinc and iron absorption, but nutritionists now think that people who habitually eat these cereals develop sufficient quantities of the enzyme that deals with phytic acid and so aids absorption.

Oxalic acid, found in chocolate, cocoa, plums, prunes, rhubarb and spinach, hinders the body's uptake of calcium by forming insoluble calcium oxalate, a complex that may contribute to kidney stones and rheumatism. Pasteurisation of milk destroys the enzyme phosphotase required for its complete absorption. Recent research has also shown that vitamin C helps iron absorption, so the iron from eggs and other foods is more likely to be utilised if an orange or some orange juice is included at the same meal.

Fats and fried food

Fried food is difficult to digest and can be a contributory cause of gastric ulcers. Depending upon the amount of fat involved in the cooking, the foodstuff under a crisply fried coating cannot be worked upon by the digestive juices – in the mouth in the case of starches such as potatoes, or in the stomach in the case of proteins such as fried fish. Saturated fats – those that are solid at room temperature – have a higher proportion of hydrogen either occurring naturally or as the result of processing, and these are not as easily utilised as softer, less processed fats or oils, which are unsaturated. Saturated fats are also more likely to be stored as body fat.

All fats and fatty foods contain both unsaturated and saturated fatty acids in varying proportions – even butter contains some unsaturated fat and since it is a relatively unprocessed product compared to many oils and margarines, it may well prove to be the more nutritious. Only those margarines or oils that specifically claim to be cold-pressed and contain linseed, safflower, sunflower, soya, peanut or corn (maize) retain the essential fatty acids needed for cell structure. They are normally only available from health food shops and do not always have a pleasant taste so I tend to use virgin olive oil or butter. Olive oil does not contain essential fatty acids, but is only harmful if an excess results in an undesired increase in weight. The rest have been through a heat process that has destroyed vitamin E, known to keep the essential fatty acids intact. Fats, allowed to go rancid, will destroy the vitamins A, D, E and K in food, preventing their absorption by the intestines and creating toxic oxides in the blood. Unless these toxins are rendered harmless by the body's immune system, they will cause molecules to link together incorrectly to destroy normal cells, a factor in many diseases including arteriosclerosis (hardening of the arteries), arthritis and cancer. In order to fortify the immune system to deal with such toxins, the body needs foods that are rich in vitamin C and foods containing selenium – good sources of which are brewer's yeast, tuna, herring and wheat germ. Abnormal and weakened arterial cells, which represent the first stage in arteriosclerosis, then attract cholesterol and other substances that are deposited on the walls, thus narrowing the vessels and contributing to high blood pressure. This latter stage where blood vessels can become choked up with fatty deposits is known as atherosclerosis.

Cholesterol

Cholesterol, present in animal foods containing fats such as eggs, butter, milk and liver was once blamed for the cholesterol deposits found in arteries. But there is evidence of the disease developing in people who regularly eat a low-cholesterol diet and also evidence that some people on a high-cholesterol diet can be completely free of the disease. Moreover, the body is able to make cholesterol from starch, sugar and other kinds of fat since it is essential for making hormones, bile acids and vitamin D. In order for cholesterol to be utilised correctly, essential fatty acids and lecithin are necessary. Lecithin is found in cold-pressed oils as well as in eggs (it is destroyed when eggs are fried), liver, nuts, wheat germ and soya beans. For lecithin to function properly, the following nutrients must also be present: vitamin B6, inositol and choline (all B-complex vitamins found in wheat germ, liver and brewers' yeast); vitamin E found in wheat germ, vegetable oils and nuts; vitamin C from fruit and vegetables; and magnesium from black molasses, honey, apples, dried fruits, wheat germ, cabbage, lettuce and celery.

Cholesterol exists in the blood and organs as HDL-cholesterol (high density lipoprotein); LDL-cholesterol (low density lipoprotein) and VLDL-cholesterol (very low density lipoprotein). A high ratio of HDL to LDL and VLDL is considered desirable as a protection against atherosclerosis, arteriosclerosis and coronary heart disease. HDL can be increased by taking a vitamin E supplement in the region of 600 per day and high blood cholesterol levels can be reduced by taking at least 500 mg of vitamin C and 3 g of nicotinic acid daily.

Sugar

Other than sugar occurring naturally in fruit, sugar intake (especially refined sugar intake) should be kept to a minimum. Apart from adding unnecessary calories, sugar disturbs the balance of other nutrients and may cause a vitamin deficiency. Vitamins B2, B3 and B6, C, E and the minerals manganese, magnesium, chromium, calcium and zinc are used in the chemical process that makes the sugar available as energy. If these vitamins and minerals are not present, sugar is incorrectly metabolised. This may strain body systems and result both in excess weight and the formation of toxins that unless eliminated, contribute not only to irritability and tooth decay, but in the long term to diabetes, chronic bronchitis, rheumatism and arthritis, as well as circulatory and heart diseases.

Ironically, white sugar, with its high concentration of sucrose devoid of other nutrients, may result in low blood sugar with consequent lack of energy and feelings of tiredness. Intake of sugar is followed by an immediate burst of energy as it floods the bloodstream, but then the body's blood sugar regulator (insulin, a hormone secreted by the pancreas) comes into action to correct the balance. In the long term, if sugar intake remains high, the pancreas may become strained and cease to produce sufficient insulin, resulting in diabetes.

Artificial sweeteners

Substances such as saccharin (a derivative of coal tar) and the cyclamates contain toxic substances, which, in excess, are thought to be a contributory cause of cancer. They should be used with extreme caution (as with any substances foreign to the body). Vitamin C can nullify any toxic effects, but if it is not in sufficient supply the liver can become overloaded and eventually damaged.

Stimulants

Cravings for salt, coffee, alcohol and nicotine are linked to the maintenance of an even level of blood sugar. All of them raise the blood sugar quickly but it then drops again quickly so that the craving returns. To maintain an even blood sugar level and to avoid exhausting the pancreas and adrenal glands responsible for sugar control, it is best to avoid stimulants and instead eat regular snacks of good carbohydrate such as a wholewheat sandwich, banana, baked potato or other fruits and vegetables, or good protein such as a boiled or poached egg, sesame or sunflower seeds or plain yogurt.

Tea, coffee, cocoa and drinking chocolate – (which contains cocoa and additional sugar) and cola drinks all contain caffeine. Tea also contains theophylline, while cocoa and chocolate contain theobromine. These substances are known as xanthines and stimulate the nervous system, the heart and the kidneys, theobromine less than the others. A cup of coffee made from ground beans may contain 150–200 mg of caffeine, depending on the size of the cup and strength of the coffee (levels are several times more than from instant coffee), but even a cup of decaffeinated coffee contains 12–25 mg, together with any chemicals used to remove the caffeine. A cup of tea may contain about 100 mg and a similar amount of cocoa or cola about 50 mg. Although the tolerance of individuals varies, 500 mg of caffeine at any time may result in extreme nervousness, a feeling of 'jitteriness' or 'jumpiness' when the telephone or doorbell rings, or difficulty in sleeping. If drunk too near bedtime, there is a frequent need to pass urine, which will rob the body of valuable water-soluble vitamins and minerals. Caffeine also causes the release of cholesterol and fats into the arteries, a rapid heart beat and excess acid in the stomach that can irritate the digestive system. This irritant effect can also occur from the tannic acid in tea. Both tea and coffee reduce the availability of minerals such as calcium, magnesium, zinc and iron.

Some research studies have shown that caffeine may be related to pancreatic cancer, but this link has not yet been proved. However, the increased nervous activity caused by caffeine uses up valuable B vitamins which, if not replaced, may result in a deficiency and may also have a detrimental effect on digestion, energy production, circulation and the skin. The kidneys may eventually become irritated and tired by excessive amounts of tea and coffee so that excess liquid is retained in the body. Cola drinks (made from cocoa leaves and kola nuts) also contain artificial preservatives, colouring, cane sugar, and artificial sweeteners. For those who love ordinary tea, try letting the pot stand for not more than five minutes, then siphoning off the liquid (not down to the leaves) into a fresh pot; this may cut down some of the tannin, caffeine and theophylline. Those who love ground coffee could try the decaffeinated beans. If you find the flavour slightly less aromatic, try it on a half and half basis.

Alcohol initially appears to have a stimulating effect because it supplies quick energy and increases the peripheral circulation, but it then acts as a depressant, affecting the central nervous system. Although wine is similar chemically to the gastric juices, it can upset the chemical balance and does not suit everyone. A glass of wine may help us to relax after a hard day's work and, taken with a meal, may aid digestion in the stomach. Too much alcohol, however, may divert blood away from the digestive organs to the skin and thus slow down digestion. Alcohol can also use up valuable B vitamins and interfere with the absorption of magnesium and zinc, as well as adding calories, and cause an increase in blood fat and cholesterol.

Salt is another stimulant that can overstrain the kidneys, increase the desire for food and drink, and lead to liquid retention. Sodium chloride (common salt) is 'hidden' in many packaged and tinned foods and is often poured on to food indiscriminately. If, in a temperate climate, the body regularly obtains a supply of more than ½–1 tsp (4–5 g.) daily (from all sources), the fluid balance of the body will be disturbed. This will reduce the proportion of potassium and calcium, both essential to correct body functioning, that the body retains. Excess salt irritates the nervous system and is also thought to be a contributory cause of sinusitis, obesity, heart trouble and possibly cancer. Salt substitutes, herb or sea salts all contain other minerals besides sodium chloride and are better balanced, but even they should be used sparingly. Pepper and mustard can also irritate the digestive tract and should not be used in excess.

Smoking may also be classed as a stimulant as it releases nervous energy. Though not directly connected with food, smoking is associated with it, and some people smoke instead of eating. In recent years, people have become more aware that smoking, or being constantly exposed to other people's smoke, may produce lung cancer, heart and circulatory disease, and chronic bronchitis. Medical reports state that a smoker shortens his life by 5½ minutes for each cigarette smoked.

Nicotine, tar, cadmium and other chemicals found in tobacco are all substances foreign to the body and have to be disposed of by the body's supply of vitamins and minerals such as vitamins A, C, E, selenium and zinc and then eliminated (see complete nutrient chart). But if the body's supply of these nutrients is inadequate the following ill-effects can occur:

- An overload of toxic substances can strain the liver.
- One cigarette can burn up approximately 15–20 mg. of vitamin C and a smoky atmosphere has a similar effect.
- Smoking 20 cigarettes per day reduces the capacity of the blood to carry oxygen by 10 per cent and consequently has an adverse effect on all metabolic processes (energy supply, building, repairing and renewal of cells and the removal of waste products) that rely on oxygen.
- Nicotine acts first as a nerve stimulant that also increases the pulse rate, then as a depressant as it uses up the B vitamins and other nutrients required for a healthy nervous system.
- Nicotine suppresses the appetite and inhibits the gastric juices so that sufficient food may not be eaten or correctly digested and absorbed.

Anyone who wants seriously to give up smoking should follow the guidelines given below both before and during the initial adjustment period; a daily vitamin and mineral supplement, rich in B and C vitamins, calcium and magnesium will help to curb any cravings and will also help to build up the nervous system and counteract feelings of irritation, panic and hunger previously suppressed by smoking. A biochemic tissue salt such as Combination B will also help. Giving up cigarettes and taking a supplement will gradually stimulate the return of a normal appetite. But it is essential to chew all foods well so that they are reduced to a form the body can use, otherwise toxins will form and may remain in the body as apparent extra weight.

Avoid using sweets, chocolate and salted nuts as cigarette substitutes. In vulnerable moments, switch your concentration to slow deep breathing and consciously relax any tense muscles. A spoonful of unheated honey will give that extra 'lift' you need by raising the blood sugar almost immediately. Or you can use aerobic exercise to get an even healthier 'kick'. The above advice will also help anyone trying to overcome dependence upon alcohol. A supplement of L-glutamine, an amino acid that is converted into glutamic acid might also help since it is the only other chemical besides blood sugar (glucose) that can be used as energy by the brain.

Drug-nutrient interactions

Antibiotics, anti-depressants, sleeping pills and anaesthetics all destroy vitamins C, B6, folic acid and K, and kill off the friendly bacteria in the intestine. The bacteria should be replaced by eating live yogurt or taking probiotics. The contraceptive pill and HRT (hormone replacement therapy) can destroy vitamins E and C, B6, folic acid and the mineral zinc.

Leaving the Berkeley, summer in Amersham, and exhibiting at Olympia

The head of the beauty therapy department at the College was planning to open her own salon in Amersham and knowing that I was getting increasingly frustrated at the Berkeley managed to seduce me away to help her. She gave me complete freedom to introduce all my therapies: exercises, yoga, reflexology, massage and colour (visible light ray) therapy, but most of all needed my help with the publicity. This was not difficult because throughout my Arden days and beyond I knew all the beauty editors so was able to capture their interest and gain the publicity that attracted many clients. One in particular was the wife of George Lucas who was making the first of the Star Wars films locally. I combined two to three days in Amersham with the rest of the week doing freelance work in London and in term-time continued at the College. All this happened in the long hot summer of 1976 so it was a relief to escape the intense heat of London. I remember people praying for rain and was on a bus early in September when the first drops fell, the passengers were so relieved that they all stood up and cheered. In May 1976 when I gave in my notice at the Berkeley the directors tried to get me to stay on part-time, but I knew this would make it difficult to maintain authority in the department. At the same time, the manager confessed that the directors had discussed giving me my own exercise room following the TV series, but would now be prepared to set aside a whole suite in which I could practise my various therapies. I was sorely tempted because I sensed I would not be working in Amersham for long. But in the end decided I needed the freedom to do my own thing without the added responsibility of managing the swimming pool, sauna and massage department as well.

The premonition that my job at Amersham would be short-lived was correct as it lasted approximately four months. The owner's husband, an accountant, decided I had performed my function in helping to place the salon on the map and so my services were surplus to requirements. Without any warning I was summarily dismissed which was quite a shock. I suppressed my feelings and behaved in a civilised manner because I couldn't run the risk of losing my job at the College. As a result, I developed an enormous boil in my armpit and remember sitting in my flat one afternoon crying from the shock of my dismissal and the pain from the boil. Extra B vitamins eventually helped me deal with the boil, but in the midst of the tears, I heard a voice in my head say 'start again on another basis'. The tears stopped immediately. I jumped up, wiped my face and set off to Tottenham Court Road (the area for buying telephone equipment in that era) and bought a telephone answering machine. I knew my solution was to expand my freelance visiting service and immediately set about writing to all my old Arden and Berkeley clients. The 'important' man, Duncan, who I had met at the Berkeley owed me a favour and paid for my business cards and colourful treatment brochures and slowly I built up a business mostly by clients recommending me to their friends, but I also had help from my journalist friends.

The following spring, 1977, I exhibited at the first Festival for Mind Body Spirit at Olympia. With the help of some of my college students I set up my stall and had an exhilarating if exhausting few days chatting up the general public – a mixture of those with discerning, open minds and the great unwashed (mostly unemployed hippie types), to whom I gave free consultations with the offer of cut-price treatments and rather unwisely gave reflexology treatments with very few washing facilities available. I stimulated a lot of interest, which was hard to cope with afterwards. I ended up losing my voice because well before the exhibition closed I had been deserted by my students. Later on I was amused to find that Dave Prowse (fitness trainer and actor – Darth Vader in *Star Wars*) had picked up one of my leaflets with the heading 'Fitness is Fun' and used it as the title for a book he was writing.

Back at the College, the head of the department (salon owner) possibly from a mixture of guilt and gratitude that I hadn't breathed a word of my dismissal to the other tutors at College offered me extra work, teaching massage, which I felt duty-bound to accept as I realised it was intended as an olive branch.

I felt grateful, but in fact nearly died of exhaustion for a month or two because I was still trying to catch up with the aftermath of the exhibition.

My mother died of a stroke in May 1978. She had been on liquid reducing pills for a while and may have had the odd mini-stroke, but was found sprawled on her dining room floor by her sister who just happened to call, which was very fortunate because my mother lived alone.

Her next door neighbour told us later on, that the night before my mother collapsed they had spent the evening together and my mother commented that she felt my father was especially close that day. I'm sure he must have drawn close to help her through the transition to the next life. On the morning of her funeral I remember walking down one of the lanes in the village and heard a blackbird singing in a very persistent manner as if to alert my attention. I was convinced this was my mother's way (she had been a singer) of telling us she was all right. It was a comforting experience.

I continued at the College until 1983, during which time we were continuing to upgrade the courses until they reached degree standard. I enjoyed the challenge, especially the interaction with the students who responded well to my style of teaching. The main problem I faced was the attitude of one of the fulltime teachers who tried to undermine me by implying that my knowledge was not up to standard. I had worked hard to ensure that I was totally on top of my subject, so fortunately was able to call her bluff and the problem subsided. It took me a while to realise she must have been envious of my work experience and reputation outside the College as many of the teachers had never had a job in the outside world.

My rapport with the girls was such that if there was any spare time at the end of a lesson we often discussed life's problems together and when I shared some of my experiences they listened with rapt attention. You could have heard a pin drop! So maybe these sessions were as valuable as the lessons. I had taught at the College for nine years and in my final year the work had become repetitive and no longer presented any challenges so I decided to wait until my students had safely passed their final exams and then gave in my notice.

Ronald Beasley, the Principal of the College of Spiritual Psychotherapeutics had died in 1979 and shortly after his death I 'felt' his hands on my shoulders and telling me 'there is a lot of work left to do' (the story of my life) and I slowly began to realise how I should respond. He had often urged us to 'throw away our massage table' which I interpreted as us needing to challenge clients/patients to do more to help themselves rather than relying upon the therapy. He also impressed upon us the need to avoid organisations with fixed dogmas, -isms and -ologies which might prevent us from being independent thinkers free to consider new truths and evolve at our own pace. Having come originally from a non-conformist (Methodist) background and having increasingly moved away from conventional thinking to find my own answers, I responded wholeheartedly to this message and am happy to think of myself as a free spirit or spiritual nomad.

Starting after Mr Beasley's death I slowly began collecting together everything learned and experienced in the field of health and healing and over the next few years spent all my free time writing, putting all my information into a 'magnum opus'. This provided me with an acceptable reason to give the College for leaving the job. Quite truthfully, I needed more time to complete the massive task I had set myself.

Along the way, I continued to work with journalists and one day was asked to make a contribution to a health and beauty book which led to me meeting an editor/packager (someone who produces books and sells them on to a publisher for distribution) who eventually became a fully-fledged publisher. This lady gave me lots of encouragement but was slow to take action and when the book was finally ready for publication, the company went bankrupt, coinciding with changes in the publishing world and the type and size of books being published. The appetite for large books diminished with the result that I was never able to find another publisher. Having been far ahead of my time I became yesterday's news almost overnight.

A year after Ronald Beasley's death I attended several weekend study courses at the College where the resident naturopath/osteopath taught techniques such as simple osteopathic manipulations, lymphatic drainage and reflexology within the magnetic aura. This involves holding the thumb within ½–1 inch from the foot being treated. Whenever I have practised this the benefits seem to be subtly different from the norm. An 'electric spark' often seems to pass between the operator and recipient indicating the transmission of energy, but is only of value if the recipient is aware of this possibility.

Developing my therapy and teaching practice

A part from working to complete my magnum opus, leaving the London College of Fashion in May 1983 enabled me to concentrate full time on my home visiting service. It was never a conscious aim, but at each step along the way I simply remember responding to opportunities that would increase my skills and sense of fulfilment.

I am pausing at this point in my story to explain how the philosophy I had adopted during my search for whole health (mental, physical, spiritual) has been the strongest influence on the way I have conducted all aspects of my life for almost fifty years, including my choice of therapies to practice when I eventually launched my home visiting service. During my final year at Barts and before going to Elizabeth Arden, I had overcome my physical fitness problems and enjoyed passing on what I had learned to clients and any interested friends. My mantra became: think right, eat right and move right (i.e. adopt positive and balanced mental attitudes, a nutritionally balanced diet and an exercise plan to suit individual needs). Not content to stop there, I was constantly seeking methods for self-help and understanding, which had led me to biochemic tissue salts, an in-depth study of vitamin and mineral supplements, reflexology, colour therapy and yoga, also such tools for such self-understanding as numerology.

After benefiting myself from these therapies and tools, I assimilated them naturally into my work. As I have mentioned earlier in the book, my continuing search for answers to life's deeper mysteries including my own relationship problems finally led me to the College of Spiritual Psychotherapeutics where I eventually realised that my destiny in this life was increasing unlikely to include marriage and children, which I had always longed for. Perhaps this was partly because of my emotional immaturity that had resulted in my spending too long in my relationship with Dennis and possibly mishandling the relationship with Jack. In any event I felt my future lay in the field of health and healing. Once I accepted this as my path to fulfilment and let my soul rather than my emotions take charge of my life, notwithstanding the obstacles and crises that beset us all, I have been blessed with a sense of inner peace.

The therapies I chose to practice are a true expression of my beliefs and are all in harmony with each other. Reflexology, yoga, colour therapy even biochemic tissue salts, work through the body's subtle energy vibrations and together with exercise and nutrition revitalise body, mind and spirit. They are all practical to use and require little or no equipment thus simplifying my operation of a home therapy service. Here is a favourite affirmation of mine, which expresses in a nutshell what I believe life is all about and is a useful reminder of how we can facilitate our journey towards wholeness:

> *Let/May my soul direct my appetites*
> *Let/May my soul direct my emotions*
> *Let/May my soul direct my heart*
> *Let/ May my soul direct my intellect*
> *Let/May my soul direct my intuition*
> *Let/May my soul finally unite with all*
> *parts of my nature to merge with spirit*

My practice developed gradually, mainly through word-of-mouth recommendations. I acquired a variety of European and American (very few English) clients and eventually my clientele extended to Iranians, Iraqis, a Qatar family, Palestinians, Greeks, Egyptians and, most of all, a host of Lebanese. I had always thought of myself as a citizen of the universe so maybe that is why I had attracted such a diverse range of nationalities including a mixture of religions, which was never a problem as my belief system (devoid of dogma) is inclusive of everyone. I particularly remember thinking how like the English in outlook some of the Palestinians were, possibly because the women were brought up to take education seriously and have a career (probably the influence of the British Protectorate in Palestine prior to 1948). The Lebanese ladies on the other hand having had an influence from the French, were on the surface more sophisticated, interested in the café society and the good life, but open-minded, generous to a fault, warm hearted and very emotional.

As the years went by, the Lebanese (mostly ladies) formed the bulk of my clientèle. I also had a good rapport with the Greeks, who are similar in some respects to the Lebanese, but less emotional, maybe the influence of the English education that many of them had received.

My introduction to the Lebanese came indirectly through an American lady, a member of one of my yoga classes, whom I massaged on a regular basis. She introduced me to a healer with undoubted abilities – a Welshman who pretended to be Japanese because he taught martial arts and was something of a megalomaniac in his family life. He was quick to impress me with his psychic abilities and after judging that my massage was satisfactory recommended me to some of his patients. There was one couple, the husband French and the wife Iranian, who were anxious for a baby, but she was having difficulties conceiving. The healer thought that massage and reflexology might help them to release deep-seated tensions. They were a delightful couple and whether or not my treatments had anything to do with it, the wife did become pregnant much to their great joy. As a result she recommended me to a Lebanese friend who recommended me to another and so on, until I eventually became known to the majority of the Lebanese community in London, who had all fled from the civil war in their country. For some reason I had an innate understanding of these ladies, many of whom were young enough to be my daughters. They were hungry for whatever I could teach them about a healthy life-style, relationships and life in general. It was a match made in heaven.

Three special ladies

In many ways the 1970s through to the early 1990s proved to be the most rewarding period for my work. There were three Lebanese ladies with whom I worked at an especially deep level. They were all passing through life-changing experiences at the time and will forever remain very dear friends although they no longer live in England.

Their faith in me was humbling and they knew they could trust me with their confidences. Suffice to say, one of them recovering from a serious riding accident was told by her specialist that she would be unlikely to ever regain her sense of taste, which she did; mainly we think as a result of the reflexology treatments.

Another lady who was having a difficult pregnancy asked for a 'healing' which involved me placing one palm within an inch or so of her abdomen and the other in the same place on her back, when she experienced a great warmth and the baby moved to a more comfortable position. Afterwards, she touched my hands and screamed because they were actually ice-cold, thus demonstrating that in this form of 'healing' it is not the therapist's energy that is used. The therapist is the channel through which the healing energy passes.

The third lady in this group was able with my help and encouragement to overcome an illness by entirely natural means without the need of medical drugs. Biochemic tissue salts played a prominent role in her recovery. Later she stepped out of the comfortable social zone that most of the Lebanese ladies lived in, to take a long, gruelling course to become a fully qualified psychotherapist. Her belief system matched my own and were it not for the fact that she was fully committed to her training and family responsibilities, I might not have fallen under the spell of the Panamanian lady yet to be mentioned. But then I would have missed a big learning curve.

The Lebanese lady, Nada, was a believer in meditation and healing and one day when she knew I was particularly exhausted, without telling me, sent me absent healing. I was sitting on a bus at the time when I felt myself engulfed in a warm comforting and re-energising heat from top to toe. I guessed it came from her and confirmed it when I telephoned her on my return home. For anyone who is open to a belief in reincarnation, Nada was in London in the spring of 2008, when we found we had both discovered the concept of sacred contracts. I had been introduced to the idea by a medium who specialises in helping people find their life purpose. In short, it is a pre-birth 'contract' willingly entered into by one or more souls (with the aid of an evolved spirit) to fulfil specific aims or make appropriate recompense for errors made in a past life. I have always felt I was 'meant' to work with the Lebanese as in my experience when we follow our destiny there is often a special sense of fulfilment and of being in the right place at the right time. But this concept became much clearer to me when I was told by two different mediums that I had once lived in Phoenicia (ancient name for the Lebanon), but had let my country folk down and had contracted to make amends in this life.

Healing, colour and Katie

During this period I was still attending courses at the College of Spiritual Psychotherapeutics and recall practising a healing/chakra balancing technique on another student that involved placing my hands over (not on) her eyes. Afterwards she experienced a definite improvement in her eyesight which I believe was in part due to our raised expectancy in the spiritually-charged atmosphere of the College. After my experience at the 1977 Festival for Mind Body Spirit, I attracted clients who were open to the possibilities of colour healing (using specific visible light rays projected through a lamp) and again I had positive results. In my experience, the recipient does not need to understand the process but must be open-minded otherwise a negative mental attitude may prevent the healing energies from entering the body. One of these clients was a psychic who said she could 'see' doctors from the spirit world overseeing my treatments. I was aware that a healing session had a different atmosphere, but never saw the spirit doctors myself. What often happened when I gave a meditative-type treatment was that I would hear myself making a totally unpremeditated comment that the client would remark answered a deep-seated need that I knew nothing about. At such times these words seemed to come through me not from my conscious mind. This kind of experience was quite frequent when a few years later I worked with recovering addicts and alcoholics who were following the 12-step recovery programme. They were very open to the type of therapies I practised.

Around the time of the Festival I read in a copy of *Here's Health* that Katie Boyle, the well known television personality and journalist was to write an article on colour therapy, which she confessed to knowing very little about, so I grasped the opportunity and decided to come to her rescue. I rang her up and she accepted my offer to share my knowledge. This resulted in several enjoyable sessions in which we established a great rapport and led to her comment that I was very persuasive. As a consequence she gave me lots of encouragement and in her article in the April 1977 edition of *Here's Health*, she described how during a bout of bronchitis, the colour therapy treatment eased the tightness in her chest and relaxed her sufficiently to fall into a deep sleep.

Working with the rich and famous

I witnessed history in the making in 1979 when I was giving a treatment in the Belgravia home of the then Chairman of the Conservative Party. Whilst downstairs the strategy of Margaret Thatcher's first victory was being planned, upstairs the lady of the house was trying to persuade me to vote for them. I was yet to be convinced so at that election I still voted Liberal (when Liberals were Liberals – long before the party became Liberal Democrats).

Around this time I was working with clients at a Palestinian household and discovered that Yasser Arafat was staying incognito in their home! I was also introduced to the Fayed family by a girl I had worked with at Elizabeth Arden's. She had been the family's masseuse, but was leaving London to get married. This was before Mohammed (the eldest of three brothers and then known as Michael) and the next brother, Ali, were married. I remember being struck by the dark, heavy Egyptian style of their interior decorations and furniture. Later on when Mohammed married Heini, a Finnish girl, and Ali married an English girl, Tracey, the wives' influence had a lightening and brightening effect on the entire apartment. I discovered that Mohammed was very generous, had a great sense of humour and had an individual way with words (as most of this country witnessed in recent years).

Tracey became a regular member of one of my yoga classes, which she enabled us to hold in one of their apartments and I continued to see Heini until after her fourth child was born in 1987, when subsequently she spent more time with the children in the country. I once massaged Dodi Fayed when he was about twenty years old and remember treating Adrianna, the Italian wife of the third brother when she was in London on 28 July 1981, the day before Charles and Diana's wedding. Little could we have foreseen the role the Fayed family would play in the events of Princess Diana's untimely death in August 1997.

Within the last few years some of my Lebanese clients met Heini at a function in the Egyptian Embassy in London. My name must have been mentioned because shortly after this she telephoned me and we enjoyed renewing our contact after so many years.

Throughout the 1980s numerous personalities left lasting impressions on me. To name a few, one was Patrick Holford an enthusiastic young man, fresh from studying nutrition with some of the best brains in America. I became one of the first distributors of his collection of naturally produced vitamin and mineral supplements. Patrick went on to open his Institute of Optimum Nutrition in London in 1984, and became one of Britain's leading spokespersons on nutrition and health issues as well as having written numerous books on nutrition. Two of his best known are *The New Optimum Nutrition Bible* published in 2004 by Piatkus Ltd and *Optimum Nutrition for the Mind* first published in 2003, also by Piatkus.

Another impressive person was Lady Lothian, one of the founders of the Women of the Year lunch held annually in the Savoy Hotel. For many years she was the president and invited fascinating and sometimes controversial women to speak at the lunch. Lady Lothian became a client of mine through our mutual hairdresser and we enjoyed many free-spirited conversations. She identified herself as a Christian feminist stoutly believing in the mother's central role in the family and was deeply concerned with human rights issues. She kindly invited me to the Women of the Year lunch which I attended for some years, meeting exceptional women from many walks of life, including well-known actresses and journalists some of whom I had already worked with at Elizabeth Arden and the Berkeley Hotel. Among the memorable speakers who addressed us were Coretta King (widow of Martin Luther King) and Valentina Tereshkova, the Soviet astronaut.

In this group of personalities was an exotic Panamanian girl who was not quite what she seemed to be, but I failed to read the subtle signs because of an emotional need of mine that she must have identified and decided to satisfy. I met her at the Grosvenor House Park Lane gym where I was teaching a yoga class. Coincidentally, Dave Prowse (Darth Vader in *Star Wars*) also used the gym at the time. The Panamanian girl, an attentive and conscientious member of the class, made quick progress and became my most proficient student, which prompted me to invite her to join one of my well-established classes. She showed a greater interest in my philosophical and natural health beliefs than any other associate had ever done so that I no longer felt mentally isolated. We even considered entering a business partnership to open a natural health centre which had always been my aim.

She was married to an attractive, fair-haired Englishman who purported to be a successful entrepreneur, but socially had a light-hearted, slightly flippant manner, a perfect foil for her dark, sophisticated, slightly mysterious persona. I later discovered they used these differences to their advantage. They were both well-liked by my other clients and only one or two ever suspected there might be something awry. One lady commented how odd it was that the girl always came to yoga classes in couture clothes, which seemed incongruous and out of place given the underlying spiritual nature of yoga. She did in fact come from a wealthy Panamanian family whom I later discovered funded her extravagant lifestyle, but it was not until she offered to lend me a dress for an evening event that I realised something was not quite right. I was to help at a charity event organised by Lady Lothian and did not have anything suitable to wear, so I called at the Panamanian lady's house (when she happened to be out) and was shown her extensive wardrobe by her husband. There were cupboards and cupboards stocked with high quality clothes, far more than she could ever use because I knew they led a fairly quiet social life. I was shocked and sickened by this display and realised that at the very least she was a shopaholic and said as much to the husband. He agreed. They both encouraged friends to make light-hearted criticisms of the one to the other. In retrospect I think it was a clever ploy to deflect any criticism of them as a couple. Suffice to say I declined the offer of one of her dresses and bought my own. In any case, even though we were the same size, our colouring was so different that none of her outfits would have suited me.

Eventually the couple presented me with a plausible story and asked for my help. The husband had done a big business deal, but there was a temporary problem with access to the money and they had a substantial bill to pay by a certain date. They knew I had recently sold a property (left to me by my father) and that I would shortly have to pay Capital Gains tax. I lent the money, they signed an IOU and agreed to repay well ahead of the date I was due to pay the tax. But this they did not do and the story became even more complicated. I began to smell a rat remembering that on the way to the bank to withdraw the loan, I became aware of a very strong vibrational pressure on my solar plexus area that in retrospect was trying to alert my attention and stop me in my path. Foolishly I ignored the warning as I felt I had to keep my promise. Readers, ignore your intuition at your peril! Ironically I was able to help a hotel reclaim money they were owed from the lady's mother. Unfortunately, the mother ignored my own request for payment and in spite of obtaining a High Court judgement against them I was never repaid a penny. In the process I discovered they had many debts, that the husband had no job, had originally been her hairdresser and, to top it all, she had tried to ruin my character with my clients. As with the problem with the couple in the Amersham Beauty Salon I kept my silence over my problems with the Panamanian lady until long after they had left England for Panama. By then, any client who might have had their doubts about me realised that I was not the guilty party.

Other interesting clients at this time included Nathan Milstein, the renowned violinist, also Ivan Lendl's in-laws and Stan Smith of Wimbledon fame.

Endings, beginnings
and the fulfilment of a dream

Apart from being one of my busiest decades, in the 1980s, I experienced a series of endings and new beginnings in my working life, the most significant beginning being the birth of a baby girl in Cape Town on 13 January 1980 that I remained ignorant of for twenty-five years. Unbeknown to me she was destined to become my main helpmate in the production of this book. Without her inspiration and encouragement it would never have happened.

My private practice continued to expand in the Kensington and Chelsea area so I decided to move closer to my clients to avoid unnecessary travelling. I eventually found a flat in the Notting Hill area close to where I had lived during the Dennis period.

Once I had moved I realised I still had a few negative memories that lingered from that period which I felt the need to confront. I re-visited the entire episode in my mind and was able to understand more fully why I had attracted the relationship and was then able to release the memories once and for all.

I reached so-called retirement age (60) in March 1987 with no intention of retiring. Nada, one of my Lebanese clients, arranged a surprise party for relatives, friends and clients which included a Tarzan-o-gram (the young man had been a contestant on Cilla Black's Blind Date television show and was later to be the first contestant on the show to marry his date). My erstwhile publisher was also invited and the guests, sympathising with me for all the delays put her on the spot and asked when the book would be published. As a reflex action probably, she answered August. As a further possible embarrassment to her, a cake had been made in the shape of the proposed book cover and she and I together cut the first slice. Motherly and friendly though she was, everything moved at a snail's pace. I had to push for an illustrator who was brilliant, also an editor and even found someone to make a promotional video, but before the end of the decade the company went bankrupt and I was the last to be told.

Later in 1987 I saw the artist for the last time (to date) when he was on a brief visit for a family wedding. He had previously urged me to let him know if ever I moved from my previous address and, with some difficulty, I managed to track him down just days before he was to 'cross the pond'. We managed to spend a few precious hours together, only to find he had just begun a new relationship with a younger woman, his marriage having ended in divorce some years earlier.

Vitality 2000 and my love affair with sunflowers – symbols of health and vitality

Sunflowers
The blossoms of good judgement and common sense. They thrive where others do not try. (Anon)

In the early 1990s, having decided on a period of mourning for all my past losses (father, mother, love of my life, sections of my manuscript that 'represented' the children I never had, etc.), I was introduced to a fantastic girl, Cassandra, with an Apple-Mac computer who helped me re-arrange my manuscript into self-work manuals under the rather grand title of *Vitality 2000, the Mary Perigoe-round of Joyful Living!* I eventually distributed them amongst my clients, but despite the fact that I think there is a certain admiration for my so-called accomplishment very few people have ever read beyond the first few pages. In this age of press-button solutions I was too readily available to answer any of their questions.

Quite apart from their nutrients – rich seeds, packed fully of vitality – sunflowers have figured prominently in my life ever since I caught my first glimpse of them many years ago when speeding through Europe in a train. Inspired by the sight of fields of giant sunflowers standing to attention like a magnificent army showing allegiance to their master, the sun, it is not surprising that I placed sunflowers in pride of place on my manual covers.

I constantly over-extended myself and remember one occasion when I succumbed to the mother of all colds. My immune system had in any case been weakened by the stress I had experienced dealing with the aftermath of the problem with the Panamanian lady. Not only did I lose my voice, but I also suffered copious nosebleeds, one of which started when I was out shopping. I dashed into a chemist shop for some tissues and the pharmacist, after pressing a box into my hands, produced a chair and a bucket and ordered me to sit down with my head in the bucket and my fingers pressed correctly on the nose to stem the flow of blood. The blood refused to stop flowing and to my horror I heard the pharmacist call for an ambulance. The shock of seeing the ambulance driver with a stretcher stopped the bleeding in a flash. At the hospital a nurse cleaned my blood-stained face and took my pulse, but it was not until several hours later that a doctor appeared. All he said was, 'You can go home now.' I was taken aback thinking the least I could expect was some kind of examination and a diagnosis. So, in an effort to get a response, I dared to suggest that perhaps the pressure on fragile capillaries could have caused the nosebleed. Without any further explanation he agreed with me. So, after having wasted most of the day in Casualty, and slightly deflated at having to make my own diagnosis, I went home. Since then, I've made every effort to avoid a recurrence and have taken more care to balance each twenty-four hours with eight hours work, eight hours leisure and eight hours rest and sleep. I've tried to eat far more fruit and vegetables (as far as possible 500 g of each) plus take a supplement of 1–2 g vitamin C with bioflavonoids daily. Although I still get one or two colds a year (a life-long weakness of mine) they are not as frequent or severe, lasting approximately five days only instead of two to three weeks. At such times I take a gram of vitamin C every three hours or so, together with Combination J from the biochemic tissue salt range and Bryonia, a homoeopathic remedy (as a cough syrup or tablet).

Within this period, apart from losing my publisher and producing my self-work manuals, my two nieces had their children, making me a great aunt six times. The birth of the first child had a dramatic affect on me. It may have been the universe's way of helping me to check that I had fully come to terms with not experiencing motherhood. After hearing my niece had given birth to a son, I was overwhelmed by a feeling of intense joy and a strong empathy with her as if I was experiencing the miracle of birth by proxy.

I also met again a gay friend I had lost touch with in the early 1980s. He had recently moved into the same area and told me he had been an alcoholic for many years, but had managed to hide it from most of his friends. Finally, he had faced up to his problem, joined Alcoholics Anonymous and become a carer for a gentleman in a local care home. After a while, it became clear to both of us that there was a role for me to play with some of the recovering alcoholics and addicts who were amongst his friends, some of whom were HIV-positive and one or two who were already suffering from full-blown AIDS. In addition to continuing with my private clients for most of the decade I worked mainly on a voluntary basis with a number of these people who were seriously committed to their 12-step recovery programme. My friend hand-picked those he thought I could help return to life in the real world. Most of them had hit rock bottom and were attempting to rebuild their lives on a step-by-step basis. They came from every stratum of society, but what I found refreshing was their complete contrast with my other well-heeled clients who were all cushioned by a comfortable lifestyle and enjoyed the support of family and friends.

According to their individual needs, I was able to use all my therapies and counselling skills, working with the recovering addicts individually or in small groups, whichever seemed appropriate. Those who could made a small financial contribution to a fund that I used to provide vitamin and mineral supplements for those who needed them. I admired their searing honesty and total commitment to their recovery. In turn, I think they appreciated my positive non-judgemental, free-thinking approach to life without attachment to any -isms or -ologies, all of which contributed to an easy rapport between us. They were convinced I was one of them, even though I had never smoked or been an addict. We shared a similar emotional make-up and I think my stability and belief in self-responsibility gave them confidence in me. For my part, I practised their number one priority of living in the day and later I was able to live literally in the moment, which is an amazingly stress-free place to be. I found that it made life more enjoyable on every level. Before this experience, I think I had often swung between the two extremes of living in the past or the future. Sadly, my gay friend died of an incurable lymphoma in the early years of the new century by which time most of the recovering addicts I had worked with had found their feet and moved on.

Fulfilling a long-held dream

When my brother-in-law retired from farming in 1998, he and my sister moved into our family home in Northiam, East Sussex, which had been rented out since my mother's death in 1978. The following year my sister, brother-in-law and myself, were finally able to fulfil a long-held dream to trek in the Himalayan region of Central Asia. We were attracted to a particular trek advertised as moderate (later revised to vigorous) to Kazakhstan and Kyrgystan in the region of the Celestial Mountains (Tien Shan). I had always felt an affinity with the mountainous region of the Himalayas, sensing that I may have lived a life in that part of the world and was probably looking for a spiritual experience. These countries had only recently opened up to tourism, following the break up of the Soviet Union, which was part of the attraction for us. The Celestial Mountains (Tien Shan) border China and are an extension of the Greater Himalaya. The area is closely associated with the Great Silk Road.

Our adventure began with a flight to Almaty in Kazakhstan and we trekked for eleven days in all, mostly six hours a day, over fairly rough terrain (with a two-day break in a base camp after eight days). We passed through a mountain range of Alpine scale along valleys, through meadows rich with wild flowers, once visiting a nomad camp and across an impressive pass. I was the eldest in the group (72 at the time) so this factor, plus my shortness of stature was probably why our leader sometimes summoned a horse to carry me the final stretch to our camp site. This was a mixed blessing as there was no saddle which made it a very uncomfortable ride, and hoisting me on and off the horse caused much amusement. The horse also carried me over the steepest part of the mountain-pass where a false step by the horse or the man leading him would have sent us all hurtling to a certain death. Strangely, I wasn't frightened, I felt I had the protection of a spiritual presence. The highlight of the trek was a wildly exciting helicopter flight (a large old Soviet Army machine that carried 25 of us) to a glacier of over 14,000 feet where we could view two of the most beautiful mountains in the world, Peak Popeda, 24,406 ft/7,439 m and Khan Tengri, 22,798 ft/7,101 m (in the same class as the Matterhorn) its upper half is of marble. En route we passed scarily close to the mountains and the sight of debris from crashed helicopters scattered over the slopes did not exactly inspire our confidence in either the machine or the pilot. The trek came to a close on return to Almaty. Before returning home we flew to the neighbouring country of Uzbekistan to visit Tashkent and especially Samarkand as we felt we were unlikely to visit this exotic area again. The people mostly wore traditional dress and seemed more conservative than their neighbours. Nevertheless, they were very friendly. The city reflected its rich history and association with Alexander the Great, Genghis Khan and Tamerlane who made it his capital.

The year of the trek (1999) Duncan, my businessman friend found himself in a difficult position financially. Never one to consider retirement, he had taken on a job in his late seventies of restoring the failing fortunes of a famous business in Norwich, only to discover that owing to the questionable behaviour of certain directors there was a shortfall in the employees' pension fund. As Chairman, he felt honour-bound to rectify the matter and I understood that, as none of the other directors were prepared to help, he made good the shortfall with his personal money. But for a large, unexpected tax bill, he might have averted disaster. As it was he had to sell his home, many of his possessions and bought a rundown property to develop and eventually sell at a profit to enable him to repay most of his debts. Before this could happen he encountered endless problems with builders and specialised materials that brought him to the brink of bankruptcy. This took a serious toll on his health, already weakened by maturity-onset diabetes that had damaged his heart and resulted in a triple by-pass operation. I was so concerned that his altruistic act had brought him to this point that I offered financial help, which he accepted (I had recently cashed in an investment plan that had reached maturity). He will remain the most positive person I've ever known and am sure that he had every intention of repaying the loan. Unfortunately, during a brief period when he could have done so, he suffered a severe stroke from which he never recovered.

My last contact with him was in December 2002 when he phoned from what must have been a hospital. His voice sounded strange which made me suspect a stroke. He just managed to ask me to visit when the phone went dead. Much to my regret I was never able to trace the call and in spite of ringing all the major hospitals, I never found him. In the spring of 2003, an uncle who had known him in business rang to say he had seen the death notice in a paper that described him as a 'spectacular enthusiast'. I had feared the worst having heard no more from my friend and immediately set about trying to find where he had died and the cause, which helped me recover from shock and channel my grief. Eventually, I tracked down the registrar who had recorded the death and obtained a copy of the death certificate which revealed the cause, the hospital in which he died, also his last home address. This information enabled me to contact his family and request repayment from his estate. Unfortunately, I was informed by the solicitor that he had left no money or assets. In spite of having all the necessary proof of the loan I was never repaid even in part. Friends thought I'd been the victim of another 'con' but I have never thought so. No pressure was put on me and I lent the money willingly. I have never regretted what I did, but felt the need for more information and decided I owed it to myself to do everything possible to reclaim some of the loan. I employed private investigators who uncovered important information, but nothing that pointed the finger at my friend. I spoke to past employees of the Norwich company and engaged a solicitor, also the police, who agreed there were suspicious circumstances around the problems with the pension fund, but insufficient evidence to bring a case. So, I have let the matter drop, knowing that I did all I could to bring the matter to a satisfactory conclusion.

Referring to my previous mention of sacred contracts, I was informed recently by two different mediums that the business friend and I had been married in a previous life and had a daughter whom we neglected because of our closeness and that prior to entering this life we had both made a contract to make amends. Hence, he married the daughter in this life (a stunningly beautiful lady) and I unwittingly helped provide her with a house she was able to sell at a profit after his death. Without my money I doubt that this would have been possible. So, mad as some readers may think me, I have found satisfaction in this belief.

During the early years of this century several people I knew in my university years re-surfaced, some of whom were writing their life story to pass on to their family. It seems to be a natural tendency to reflect on one's life experiences in later life. In trying to trace me, one of these friends, a woman, came across Jack, the artist who had also lost my address and wanted to find me. She found me through a Canadian relative of the same surname and told Jack, and he and I renewed contact in December 2006.

In the summer of 2001, Mark, a Methodist Minister from Cape Town sent an e-mail to my sister to say he was coming to England for a sabbatical and would like to visit us and discover more about his family's roots. Mark's father, also a Methodist Minister, Charles Stephenson, was my father's second cousin and his mother came from our locality. We met Mark at the local station, brought him home for a late breakfast and spent a busy day showing him where some of his relatives had lived, and generally getting to know each other. And that brings me back to the baby girl born in 1980 – Mark is her father.

Reflections on delaying the ageing process

It is now more than fifty years since I vowed to try and slow down the ageing process naturally, and to date I'm reasonably satisfied with the outcome. My weight and shape have remained stable, and my hair, in spite of an increasing number of grey hairs, has so far retained much of its own colour and happily my hairdresser assures me I won't go bald. I have successfully relied on herbal and homeopathic remedies, including biochemic tissue salts and vitamins and mineral supplements to overcome common ailments and so far have managed to avoid serious illness. On the down side I need reading glasses, have lost roughly two to three centimetres in height and had signs of arthritis in both hips (recently rectified by successful hip replacements). I believe my arthritic condition had been aggravated by the stressful aftermath of Duncan's demise and when I had several falls in quick succession.

Most of us would like to delay the ageing process and prevent the onset of serious disease even though we may not be obsessed with the search for the elixir, pill or implant to make us 'eternally young'. We may envy those who have developed an inner serenity which makes them seem younger in spite of facial lines and grey hairs. Their response to life's challenges has made them more tolerant, wiser and increasingly confident in the spiritual truths they have discovered and come to live by. They have found their true selves by discarding layers of 'dead wood' in the form of faulty mental and physical attitudes, and have emerged lighter in spirit and body and filled with boundless enthusiasm for life. Surely this is the secret of eternal youth?

I believe that it is we ourselves who determine consciously or subconsciously the rate at which we age. As I've grown older I have realised that it has less to do with luck, circumstances or heredity than our ability to sustain or increase our enthusiasm for life. This in turn makes us seek positive solutions to problems, nurture realistic ambitions, and have gentler reactions to stressful situations which we are then able to channel creatively.

Some people say we are entirely what we eat, and slavishly follow the latest 'rejuvenation' diet. Alexis Carrell of the Rockefeller Institute in America, during laboratory experiments with living cells, highlighted the importance of essential nutrients and oxygen when he concluded that' tissue cells are essentially immortal; give cells all the essential nutrients they need, remove promptly all wastes and poisons and they can be kept alive indefinitely'. We can, however, still poison our body chemistry by bitter thoughts. Severe shock or prolonged physical or emotional exhaustion can slow down the building of healthy new cells and the removal of dead ones. The same is true of too little sleep on a regular basis, since cell repair and renewal take place during sleep. Many people swear they can hold onto youth through aerobic exercise because every cell can be strengthened and oxygenated, but such exercise must always be graded carefully, and we still have to supply the correct nutrients in food.

In the further pursuit of youth, those who can afford it may prefer cosmetic surgery. In the case of facelifts and the removal of body fat, however, unless future habits are radically changed, the procedures may have to be repeated. Some years ago cell therapy injections based on ribonucleic acids (RNA), extracts of cells from unborn animals, were popular. Such treatments may have prolonged the lives of famous people such as Sir Winston Churchill, Somerset Maugham, Charlie Chaplin and the Duke of Windsor, to name but a few, but did not prevent degenerative diseases.

Nowadays many people swear by supplements such as royal jelly, ginseng or vitamin E. Yet others regularly use collagen fillers or botox injections to plump up the facial skin and special external treatments including herbal clay masks or the latest skin creams, hoping to increase the speed and efficiency of cell regeneration, as the manufacturers claim.

Free radicals and other chemical agers
Research has produced a theory formulated by Johan Bjorksten known as chemical cross-linking. This is an oxidation process in which molecules link

together to form undesirable chemical bonds which interfere with normal cell structure. It can affect proteins such as collagen in the skin, body lipids or fats, or nucleic acids which make up the DNA and RNA of 'genetic material' of cells. Not only does this process cause the skin to wrinkle and lose its elasticity but it can also increase the risk of cancer, arteriosclerosis, arthritis and other degenerative diseases.

Agents held responsible for cross-linking include ultraviolet light, x-rays, ketones (incompletely metabolised fat or protein particles found in the blood of diabetics or people on high protein or low carbohydrate diets), air pollutants such as acetaldehyde (also found in cigarette smoke and produced in the liver from drinking alcohol), lead from petrol fumes, aluminium from cooking utensils, some antiperspirants and processed cheese, cadmium from coffee, tea, cigarettes or tin cans, and rancid fats and oils. All of these produce free radicals – highly reactive atoms or molecules which form toxic peroxides and cause cross linking reactions.

To counteract the risk of cross linking and generally to delay the ageing process, nutritionists recommend vitamins A, B-complex, C including bioflavonoids, and E and the minerals selenium and zinc. Individual doses are best prescribed by a doctor or other expert familiar with nutritional therapy. Some experts on ageing believe that proteolytic (protein-digesting) enzymes occurring in certain foods may have the power to reverse the effects of cross-linking. Raw papain in papaya and raw bromelain in pineapple are two examples.

Research by Richard Wurtman of the Massachusetts Institute of Technology has revealed that some of the neurotransmitters (chemical messengers) in the brain which decline as we grow older, contributing to fatigue, depression, addictions and mental illness, are dependent upon specific nutrients. Serotonin, acetylcholine and the three catecholamines (adrenalin, noradrenalin and dopamine) are the neurotransmitters which are directly dependent upon diet. Serotonin, which helps the body relax and sleep, is produced from tryptophan, an amino acid occurring in, for example, eggs, milk, sesame seeds and spinach. Choline (one of the B vitamins) from such foods as liver, kidney, heart, wheat germ wholegrains, brewers yeast, vegetables and fruit along with the mineral manganese (from wholegrains, green vegetables, pineapple and nuts for example) both help in the formation of acetylcholine, a chemical that scientists believe plays an important role in memory functions, appetite control, and sex drive.

The catecholamines help regulate the sex drive (a deficiency often shows as a lack of motivation in older people) as well as the level of growth hormones. These in turn are partly responsible for the immune system (a lack may show in increased infections as well as susceptibility to faster ageing). Catecholamines are produced from amino acids such as phenylalanine (found particularly in eggs, beans, soya products and cottage cheese), L ornithine and L arginine (found in wholegrains, especially wheat germ, soya beans, cheese and eggs) stimulate the production of growth hormones.

Anti-ageing nutrients

Believing as I do that spiritual and mental energies have a stronger influence on our lives than the physical, I shall never be convinced that we can slow down the ageing process by diet alone. Nonetheless it obviously plays an important role as is proved by the number of reports of people who, through dietary means, have reversed the process of degenerative diseases such as chronic bronchitis, rheumatism and arthritis, or who experience increased energy and resistance to disease.

Scientists are continually searching for the fundamental reason why, as we grow older, more cells tend to die than are replaced. All body cells contain a set of genes made up of a molecule called DNA (deoxyribonucleic acid) which contains the blueprint for replicating that cell. Another molecule RNA (ribonucleic acid) increases the production of an energy-storing molecule called ATP (adenosine triphosphate) and assembles materials needed for repair and replacement so that they can be used according to the instructions stored in the DNA. Our bodies must replicate their DNA and RNA from food sources.

Adequate amounts of DNA and RNA can be obtained from eating such foods as brewers' yeast, liver, fish, wheat germ, lentils and dried beans.

Living foods

Only living foods, those still containing their own life force, have the power to increase our vitality. The best are those that would grow if they or their seeds were planted, for example, raw fruits and vegetables, nuts and seeds such as sunflower and sesame. Second best would be any of the above lightly cooked; also pulses (peas, beans, lentils), wholegrains (especially nutritious in their sprouted form), unpasteurised milk, if obtainable yoghurt and yogurt-cheese and other unprocessed cheeses (hygienically stored to avoid infection obtainable in France, but not legal in the UK) and from healthily reared cows. Third best would be cooked eggs, meat, poultry, fish (all healthily produced) and so on; the further the food is separated from direct sun energy, the more dead it becomes.

In parts of the world where isolated groups of people have experienced a long lifespan and low incidence of disease (Ecuador, Asia, Georgia for instance) the common factors are:
- joy in living and the acceptance that it is normal to live long and healthily;
- mountain air;
- farming or similarly active work, mainly out of doors;
- serene family and community life;
- diet of naturally grown foods, mainly fruits, vegetables and wholegrains, moderate amounts of milk and cheese and very little meat.

The living and eating habits of the Hunzas, who live high in the Himalayas now part of western Pakistan, have been much publicised. Until they were subjected to de-vitalised foods from the outside world, the Hunzas were renowned for their health, vitality and longevity. They showed no signs of strain and stress, led a natural life with an even balance between work and recreation, and lived happily together.

The Hunzas believe in three main phases of life; the young years full of excitement and yearning for knowledge, the middle years for developing poise and appreciating all the advantages of youth, and the rich years where the advantages of mellowness and tolerance are added to the qualities of the other two periods. The Hunzas are not clock watchers; they do not believe in retirement and people of 90 are still working happily.

The Hunza diet consists of brown rice, wholewheat, barley, buckwheat, millet, chickpeas, beans, lentils, fresh mainly goat's milk (which has more available calcium than cow's milk) buttermilk, leafy green and root vegetables, clarified butter, cheese, and fruit, chiefly apricots and mulberries, both fresh and sun-dried. They eat meat only on rare occasions. All their foods are largely grown and eaten within the same environment. The Bulgarians, also renowned for their longevity, put their faith in yogurt, soft cheeses and sun-ripened fruits and vegetables. Take your pick from the above suggestions if you wish to increase the quality and quantity of your years.

Most people are conditioned to associate old age with disability and disease, so the first step is to change this attitude. It is my experience that we all gradually become a living image of what we believe. Since our basic beliefs affect us mentally and physically and determine everything we do, we must continually endeavour to recognise the consequences of our day-to-day lifestyles, attitudes and habits and make positive changes before the ill effects take hold. Every situation can be overcome mentally, even if disease in the physical body has progressed too far to cure and just as we must accept responsibility for the situation in which we find ourselves, so most problems can be resolved by positive adjustments to circumstances and seeking more light.

Where do we go from here?

Reflecting on my life path so far, I can see how certain incidents that once caused me a great deal of grief, have been woven into the overall pattern and enriched the experiences that I am able to draw upon in my work and everyday life. If readers believe, as I do, that life is for experiencing and learning, I hope that if we are prepared to take responsibility for the consequences of our thoughts (motives) and actions, we are more likely to turn mistakes into opportunities for positive change. This ongoing process inevitably leads to a greater understanding of ourselves and others so that we become more integrated and at peace, both within ourselves and with the outside world. What's on the inside is reflected on the outside … what you see is what you get …

Life today is lived at an ever increasing pace, whether from choice or outside pressure, so it's small wonder that few people stop to consider seriously the effect that their attitudes and habits will have on their long-term health and happiness. Using the topical problem of obesity, as an example, it saddens me to see an ever-growing number of people of all ages growing fatter, almost by the day, apparently oblivious of the risks they are taking of developing serious disease if their habits remain unchecked.

This current problem may well be part of a greater malaise in society where many people struggle to make sense of life and find a meaningful purpose. Some may find short-term satisfaction from food or seeking fame (by almost any means) or aspiring to achieve a perfect body image as constantly portrayed in the media, neither of which solution is likely to increase a sense of self-worth or lead to lasting fulfilment.

Though seldom given the publicity they deserve, sterling work is done in some areas by voluntary groups who provide much needed support and useful activities to deprived members of their community but these organisations are often hamstrung through lack of sufficient funding.

My heart goes out especially to young people in today's world, many of whom represent the fall-out from the breakdown in social and family life, emptying churches, general disillusionment with authority figures and the current street gang drink-and-drug culture. The fundamentalist evangelical approach of some sections of Christianity, Islam, and other faith groups (not to be confused with militant extremism) does provide a strict moral framework and the established religious hierarchy acts as a kind of spiritual insurance policy or comfort blanket. To some people this safety net and feeling part of a spiritual family is preferable to the sometimes lonelier path of discovering and working with one's own personal philosophy. But enquiring minds cannot accept without question the somewhat rigid dogma of belief systems and cultural influences formulated many centuries ago. Likewise, free spirits are often deterred by the methods used to attract converts that can resemble benevolent brainwashing.

We are all at different stages on life's journey, but I hope readers have been encouraged by my story and will choose to work with my suggestions as well as continuing to explore new ideas of your own, wherever you find them – whether it be from television, the internet, discussion groups, newspaper articles, radio programmes, books, lectures and so on, weighing them up against your current beliefs. Never be afraid to drop old prejudices and embrace new truths as you discover and test them out in everyday life.

In London such organisations as the College of Psychic Studies, and esoteric bookshops like Watkins or the equivalents in your area are well worth investigating. Follow your own path by responding positively to all the challenges that life brings, and remember: we all eventually become a living image of what we wholeheartedly believe. Health is balance: balanced thought, balanced nutrition, balanced movements, balanced breath. Stagnation is Death but Light is Life and Life is Movement … so keep moving – mentally, physically and spiritually.

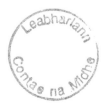

Nutrient chart

To use as a reminder of the best food sources of essential nutrients.

Many people believe that an average diet will keep them healthy, but this is not necessarily the case. Repeated dietary surveys show that the intake of several essential nutrients is deficient, for example, vitamin B6, folic acid, vitamin C, iron, magnesium and zinc.

This chart is intended as a useful checkpoint for readers confused by the constantly changing advice given in the popular press.

Nutrient	Functions	Good sources
Proteins: Made up of carbon, hydrogen, oxygen, nitrogen, sulphur and phosphorus to form amino-acids. Over 40 occur in nature but only 23 are considered vital. The 8 amino acids that the body cannot make are isoleucine, lysine, leucine, methionine, threonine, phenylalanine, tryptophan, valine. Growing children also require arginine and histidine.	Building and repairing body tissues, including haemoglobin (the iron-containing protein substance in red blood cells), hormones, antibodies and enzymes that aid energy production, digestion, building of new and breaking down of old cells.	**Complete protein:** Organ meat such as liver, heart, kidney, brain; muscle meat, eggs, fish, fowl, cheese, milk, yoghurt. **Less complete protein:** Soya beans (low in methionine otherwise complete), seeds, nuts, dried peas, beans, lentils. *Note:* 1 gram of protein = approx. 4 calories.
Carbohydrates: Made up of carbon hydrogen and oxygen (2 atoms of hydrogen to 1 of oxygen).	Provide energy for the functions of the body including muscular exertion. Assist digestion and assimilation of other foods, e.g. protein and fat.	Wholegrain bread, cereals and flour products, pulses, vegetables and fruits. Sugar as such should be unnecessary. *Note:* 1 gram of carbohydrate = approx. 4 calories.
Fats: Made up of carbon, hydrogen and oxygen (more carbon and hydrogen and less oxygen than in carbohydrates). Two main types of fat: Saturated – solid at room temperature e.g. butter, lard and margarine. Unsaturated – polyunsaturated e.g. sunflower oil or mono-unsaturated e.g. olive oil.	Provide sustained energy and heat insulation under skin. Pad and protect nerves and support internal organs. Provide medium for absorption of vitamins A, D, E, F and K. Provide material for cell structure – see Vitamin F.	Natural unheated oils and fats, including virgin olive oil. Linseed oil, safflower and sunflower oil are the best sources. Others include butter, cream, cheese and sunflower seeds. *Note:* 1 gram of fat = approx. 9 calories.

Note: The Food and Agricultural Organisation of the World Health Organisation suggest that protein intake should not fall below 1 g per 2 lb. (1 kg) body weight. Fats and carbohydrates should not fall below 1 g per 31 lbs (1½ kg) body weight. Remember that 1 g refers to pure protein, fat or carbohydrate, not to foods containing a mixture, almost all foods contain more than one nutrient. For example, an ounce of chicken (weighed raw) contains 5.9 g protein, 1.9 g fat; an ounce of butter contains 23.4 g fat, 0.1 g protein; an ounce of wholemeal bread contains 13.2 g carbohydrate, 2.7g protein and 0.9 g fat.

Nutrient	Functions	Good sources
Vitamins: **Vitamin A** Fat-soluble Note: All fat-soluble vitamins i.e. vitamins A, D, E, F and K can be stored in the liver. Chemical name, retinol also made from carotene in vegetables and fruit by the liver and can be stored in body fat. The latter form is known as beta-carotene and is half as potent as the retinol form.	Essential for growth and function of skin and mucous membranes of eyes, mouth, ears, nose, throat, lungs, genital organs and digestive tract. Helps maintain healthy glands, bones, teeth, nails, hair, eyesight and prevent dry skin. Helps liver to resist infection in body (bronchitis and other respiratory infections, allergies, hayfever).	Liver, kidney, cod, halibut, and turbot, fish liver oils, egg yolk, yoghurt, cream, milk, cheese and butter within limits. All green, yellow and orange vegetables and fruits. *Note*: Destroyed by light and air during storage and by over cooking.
Vitamin B Complex Water-soluble *Note:* All water-soluble vitamins i.e. the entire B Complex and vitamins C and P (bioflavonoids) cannot be stored in the body so it is important to get a regular supply. **Vitamin B1- Thiamine**	Essential for growth, for starch and sugar metabolism (acts as a 'wick' to oxidise them) and for energy production.	Dried brewers' yeast, yeast extract, wheat germ, liver, heart, brain, kidney, muscle meat, poultry, fish, nuts, soya beans, wholegrain cereals, bread and flour products, brown rice and molasses. *Note:* Destroyed by excessive cooking, heat, air, baking soda and preservatives.
Vitamin B2 – Riboflavin	Essential for growth, assists B1 in starch and sugar metabolism. Helps eyes to see in twilight, assists health of skin, mouth and tongue. Raises body's resistance to athlete's foot and fungal infections.	Dried brewers' yeast, yeast extract, liver, kidney, heart, wheat germ, cheese, eggs, soya flour, yoghurt, green leafy vegetables, soya beans, wholegrains and brown rice. *Note:* Destroyed by light, heat and soda.

Nutrient	Functions	Good sources
Vitamin B3 – Niacin (Also known as Nicotinic Acid, Nicotinamide or Niacinamide.)	Assists B1 and B2 in starch and sugar metabolism. Stimulates peripheral circulation, helps normal functioning of liver, brain, nervous system and soft tissues.	Same as B1 and B2.
Vitamin B5 – Pantothenic Acid (All known as Calcium Pantothenate.)	Essential for growth, normal functioning of digestive system, production of antibodies, prevention of grey hair. Assists manufacture of nerve chemicals, increases resistance to stress and production of cortisone.	Dried brewers' yeast, liver, brain, heart, nuts, wheat germ, wholewheat and oats, bran and other wholegrain products, poultry, unsulphured dried fruits, pulses, brown rice, eggs, cheese, yoghurt, broccoli and green leafy vegetables.
Vitamin B6 – Pyrodoxine	Anti-depression vitamin. Essential for the production of antibodies, the absorption of B12, necessary for healthy blood, nerves, muscles, hair and skin (can cure adolescent acne), assists in the utilisation of protein, fats and carbohydrates. Essential for the production of pancreatic enzymes, so helps prevent allergies and diabetes. Helps to balance sodium and potassium and regulate body fluids. In supplement form in conjunction with zinc is used to relieve premenstrual syndrome, liquid retention, air and seasickness, sickness in pregnancy and postnatal depression. Also helps relieve muscular cramps and impairment of colour, texture and growth of hair.	Dried brewers' yeast, wheat germ liver, molasses, lean meat, fish, oatmeal, soya flour, pulses, peanuts, pecans, seeds, bananas, avocados, green peppers, green leafy vegetables and egg yolk. *Note:* Destroyed by excessive cooking (245°F/118.3°C), air, light, oestrogens in the contraceptive pill and hormone replacement therapy, antibiotics, tranquillisers and other medicinal drugs.
Vitamin B12 – Cyanocobalamin Contains the mineral cobalt.	In conjunction with folic acid, helps build healthy red blood cells, protein, and to improve RNA production, essential for healthy nerves.	Liver, kidney, tongue, muscle meats, yoghurt, milk, eggs, dried brewers' yeast if specially bred to contain it (strepto myces griseus mould is rich in B12), blue cheese such as Roquefort which increases its B12 content by up to 15% during ripening, fermented soya bean products such as tofu or miso.

Nutrient	Functions	Good sources
Folic acid	Influences size and number of red blood cells. Essential for healthy functioning of liver and endocrine glands. One of the factors necessary for retention of natural hair colouring. Essential for brain and nerve function so critical during pregnancy for development of the baby's brain and nerves.	Dried brewers' yeast, soya flour, soya beans, wheat germ, liver, kidney, lean beef and veal, green leafy vegetables, particularly uncooked spinach, oranges, lemons and grapefruit, wholemeal bread, brown rice, eggs, bananas, cheese and root vegetables. Note: Destroyed by the oestrogens in the contraceptive pill and hormone replacement therapy, antibiotics, tranquillisers and other medicinal drugs.
Choline	Essential for healthy functioning of liver, kidneys, spleen, thymus gland and lactation. Works in association with inositol to aid correct assimilation of fat so that it is dissolved and the cholesterol does not stick to the arterial walls. Used to make acetycholine, an important nerve transmitter.	Liver, lecithin granules, kidney, heart, egg yolk, soya beans, soya flour, wheat germ, dried brewers' yeast, nuts, whole oats and wheat, citrus fruits, green leafy vegetables, green beans, bananas, root vegetables and milk.
Inositol	In association with B6 and folic acid, helps prevent thinning hair, essential for healthy functioning of heart, liver, brain and muscles. Acts as a natural tranquilliser. Works in association with choline for correct fat assimilation. Helps in utilisation of vitamin E.	Lecithin granules, liver, brain, heart, wheat germ, eggs, yoghurt, milk, wholewheat and oats, brown rice, nuts, molasses, pulses, bananas, wholewheat bread, green leafy vegetables, soya flour, soya beans, chicken, root vegetables and dried brewers' yeast.
Para-amino benzoic acid Not universally recognised. Some authorities regard it as being the same as Pantothenic acid.	Essential for healthy functioning of endocrine glands. One of the factors necessary for hair pigment along with choline and pantothenic acid and other B vitamins all of which are put out of action when the friendly bacteria in the intestines are destroyed by antibiotics and other drugs.	Can be manufactured by friendly bacteria in the intestine when butter, milk and live yoghurt is eaten. Contained in liver, brewers' yeast, wholegrain rice and other cereals, wheat germ and molasses. Lesser amounts in beef and pork.

Nutrient	Functions	Good sources
Biotin Also known as Vitamin H	Essential for normal cell growth, healthy hair and skin; healthy nervous system.	The friendly bacteria in the intestines, if present in sufficient quantities should be able to make enough for the body's needs. Contained in dried brewers' yeast, liver, kidney, fish, brown rice, soya beans and soya flour, peanuts, chicken, cheese, yoghurt and milk. *Note:* Destroyed by uncooked white of egg.
Vitamin C Water-soluble When occurring naturally in foods it is found in conjunction with bioflavonoids (see vitamin P). In its synthetic form it is known as ascorbic acid. Ascorbic acid is mildly acid in the digestive tract and a large dose (several grams) does not suit everyone, an alternative form (calcium ascorbate) is mildly alkaline in the digestive tract.	Is an essential ingredient of collagen, the protein intracellular 'glue' of the skin, connective tissue, cartilage and bone; activates while blood cells and acts as an anti-viral and anti-bacterial agent. Like vitamin E, it is an antioxidant. The ascorbic acid attaches itself to the harmful oxide and takes it out of the body. It can also deal with carbon dioxide and some pesticides in the same manner. Essential for healthy teeth, gums, capillary walls, bones and eyes. In supplement form in excess of 5000 mg can act as a laxative.	Rosehips, acerola cherries, oranges, blackcurrants, watercress, green peppers, liver, kidney, potatoes and in smaller quantities in many other fruits and vegetables. *Note:* Destroyed in cooking and by air, smoking one king-size cigarette can destroy up to 25 mg. Any shock can destroy reserves in seconds. Also destroyed by oestrogens in the contraceptive pill and hormone replacement therapy, antibiotics and other medicinal drugs.
Vitamin D Fat-soluble **Vitamin D2** Ergocalciferol plant sources **Vitamin D3** Cholecalciferol animal sources. The main active form of vitamin D)	Essential for healthy digestion, bones, teeth, and energy production, prevents and cures rickets, also used to treat tetany, psoriasis and shortsight. Helps in absorption of calcium and phosphorus primarily (so essential in prevention of osteomalacia and osteoporosis), and iron and magnesium secondarily. Helps control balance of calcium between bones and plasma. See calcium.	Fish liver oils in particular, also oily fish such as herring and mackerel; a little is contained in milk products (cream, butter, cheese, yoghurt), egg yolk, sunflower seeds and oil, also liver. The synthetic form is added to various foods such as margarine, dried milk powder and yoghurt. The sun's ultraviolet rays act on ergosterol (provitamin form) to produce vitamin D2 and on the skin to produce vitamin D3 which is absorbed into the blood stream and stored in the oil glands under the skin or in the liver.

Nutrient	Functions	Good sources
Vitamin E Fat-soluble (A complex vitamin consisting of alpha, beta, gamma, and delta tocopherols; the most effective is alpha tocopherol.)	Allows cells to function with less oxygen and keeps red blood cells supplied with oxygen so assists the function of muscles, also the prevention or cure of varicose veins, phlebitis and other circulatory problems including arteriosclerosis and coronary heart disease. Good for the skin and improves fertility. Speeds the healing of burns and wounds and impedes formation of scar tissue. It protects lungs from air pollution and, like vitamin C, it sacrifices itself to toxic oxides and so helps prevent destruction of unsaturated fats, hormones and other vitamins.	Unheated wheat germ, wheat germ oil, linseed oil, safflower oil, sunflower seeds and oil, soya beans and oil are the best sources. Also found in other unrefined (unheated) vegetable oils, nuts, including peanuts, egg yolk and brown rice. A little is found in green leafy vegetables, calves' liver, meat, milk, molasses, peas and green beans. *Note:* Anyone taking oestrogen in the contraceptive pill or hormone replacement therapy will have an increased need of vitamin E and may need vitamin E supplements.
Vitamin F Fat-soluble Essential fatty acids **Omega 3** EPA: Eicosapentaenoic Acid, DHA: Docosahexaenoic Acid **Omega 6** GLA: Gammalinolenic Acid – made in body from linoleic acid, some GLA's made into arachidonic acid.	Maintains cell membranes, pads nerve sheaths. Found in association with vitamin E which prevents vitamin F combining with oxygen in the air and becoming rancid. In the body, combines with oxygen and cholesterol to be broken down into forms used for growth, production of bile and skin health. GLA and EPA produce prostaglandins (hormone- like substances) that have an anti- inflammatory effect so helpful in reducing pain. Prostaglandins from arachidonic acid have a pro-inflammatory effect.	**Omega 3** (EPA & DHA) Mackerel, herring, tuna, salmon, sardines, linseed (flax), sunflower seeds. **Omega 6** (GLA) Evening primrose oil, safflower (borage) oil, sunflower oil, corn oil, sunflower seeds, pumpkin seeds, walnuts, wheat germ, sesame seeds, a little in butter. Some GLA is converted into arachidonic acid needed for brain cells and found in red meat. **Omega 9** Derived from oleic acid – olive oil a good source. Not an essential fat but neither is it harmful like hard fat or heated vegetable oils (see under fats) unless taken in excess which would cause an increase in body fat.

Nutrient	Functions	Good sources
Vitamin K Fat-soluble	Essential for the production of prothrombin, the blood-clotting agent.	Cauliflower, Brussels sprouts, broccoli, green leafy vegetables and liver.
Vitamin P Water-soluble Bioflavonoids, citrin hesperin and rutin.	Aids vitamin C in all its functions, but whereas vitamin C affects large blood vessels, vitamin P increases strength and permeability of small blood vessels (capillaries). Used in treatment of high blood pressure and strokes.	The same as vitamin C (but not present in synthetic ascorbic acid). Found in the flesh of fruit near the pith so can be missing in fruit juices. Rosehips, lemons, oranges, grapefruit, blackcurrants, apricots, grapes, cherries, blackberries, cabbage, plums, parsley, prunes, watercress.
<u>Minerals</u>: **Calcium**	Builds bones and teeth and helps prevent rickets, soft or porous bones (osteomalacia and osteoporosis respectively), and tooth decay. Helps prevent insomnia, promotes a healthy heart and nervous system, helps blood to clot and relieves aching muscles. Works with magnesium in the ratio of 3:2 calcium magnesium, 2:1 calcium phosphorus (which should be borne in mind if taking supplements) and vitamin D.	Milk (may not be absorbed if milk is pasteurised), yoghurt, buttermilk, cheese, almonds, pumpkin and sesame seeds (4 oz/113 g contain over 1000 mg), canned fish and pulses also prunes and figs, honey, eggs, cress, carrots, celery, cauliflower, beetroot, onions, tomatoes. *Note:* Contained in oats and other wholegrains but phytic acid, also present, can destroy it. Also contained in plums, prunes, rhubarb and spinach, but oxalic acid present can render it unavailable to the body.
Chlorine (In its natural form; i.e. not as a chemical added to water supplies.)	Acts as a purifying agent: stimulates perspiration and peristaltic movements in colon. Aids manufacture of hydrochloric acid.	Raw milk, (unpasteurised – not readily obtainable), raw egg yolk*, raw cabbage, raw carrots, spinach, asparagus, cucumber, radishes, beetroot, tomatoes, raisins.

*Since the outbreak of salmonella poisoning in 1988 the Government has recommended that raw egg and recipes containing it should be avoided.

Nutrient	Functions	Good sources
Chromium	Essential for effective carbohydrate and sugar metabolism. Helps normalise hunger and reduce food cravings. To be effective, chromium needs to be combined with vitamin B3 and three amino acids known as glucose tolerance factor (GTF: glycine, glutamic acid and cysteine) to balance blood sugar. If chromium is deficient, dizziness or irritability could occur after 6 hours without food.	Dried brewers' yeast, liver, molasses, egg yolk, beef, cheese, wholegrain, potatoes, bananas, carrots and mushrooms.
Cobalt	Needed in small amounts to help assimilate vitamin B12.	Green leafy vegetables, scallops, cod, liver, kidney and muscle meats.
Copper	Helps iron to build red blood cells. Is a constituent of enzymes and proteins. Essential to the production of ribonucleic acid (RNA) part of the nucleus of every cell.	Liver, kidney, oysters, crab, brain, seaweed (kelp), dried brewers' yeast, lecithin, wheat germ, sunflower seeds, nuts, pulses, molasses. (Presence dependent upon copper being present in the soil.)
Fluorine	Works in conjunction with calcium and silicon to strengthen teeth and bones. Calms nerves. Sodium fluoride added to water reservoirs can be a toxic by-product of industry but calcium fluoride as found in nature is not.	Cheese, milk, raw egg yolk*, wholegrains, spinach, watercress, cauliflower, leeks, Brussels sprouts, chives, raw cabbage.
Iodine	Essential for production of thyroid hormones, stimulates physical and mental energy. Increases circulation, helps prevent wrinkles and removes toxins from nervous system; helps assimilation of calcium. Too little may result in low blood pressure, easy weight gain, listlessness, anaemia and goitre.	Seaweed (kelp), Irish moss, lobster, carrots, cabbage, green beans, potatoes, artichokes, garlic, onions, leeks, tomatoes, lettuce, pineapple, strawberries, peas.

*Since the outbreak of salmonella poisoning in 1988 the Government has recommended that raw egg and recipes containing it should be avoided.

Nutrient	Functions	Good sources
Iron	Essential ingredient of haemoglobin (haem = iron, globin = protein) – the oxygen-carrier in the red blood cells and the remover of carbon-dioxide. Increases vitality and resistance to disease. Can be used again when old cells breakdown and small amounts are stored in the liver, spleen and bone marrow. Copper, vitamin C, calcium and vitamin B6 are necessary for complete iron absorption. If depleted may result in anaemia, fatigue, listlessness, loss of appetite, pale skin or sore throat.	Dried brewers' yeast, liver, kidney, beef, egg yolk, nuts, wheat germ, oats, molasses, apricots, unsulphured dried fruits, dried peas, beans, lentils, deep green leafy vegetables, beetroot and canned sardines. *Note:* Phytic acid present in wholegrain may make it unavailable to the body.
Magnesium	Works with calcium to maintain strong bones and teeth and promote healthy muscles (including heart muscles) helping them and the nerves to relax, so can ease premenstrual syndrome. Essential for energy production activates essential digestive enzymes.	Soya beans, soya flour, dried brewers' yeast, brown rice, dried peas, seeds, nuts, wholewheat and oats, green leafy vegetables, bananas, unsulphured dried fruits.
Manganese	Helps form healthy bones, cartilage and nerves. With zinc balances blood sugar, essential for reproduction and brain function, promotes healthy RNA and DNA.	Wheat germ, wholegrain, avocados, watercress, endive, parsley and other green vegetables, chestnuts, hazelnuts, almonds, pineapple, bananas, liver and eggs.
Phosphorus	Builds bones, teeth and muscle tissue. Components of RNA and DNA, helps maintain acid/alkaline balance in body. Assists metabolism and energy production.	Dried brewers' yeast, wheat germ, soya flour, cheese, brown rice, wholemeal bread, eggs, chicken, cod, beef, yoghurt, and other protein foods. Some in unsulphured dried fruits and a little in other fruits. *Note:* Too much meat, cheese, eggs and fish could upset the normal acid/alkaline balance.

Nutrient	Functions	Good sources
Potassium	Essential for the building of tissues, in conjunction with calcium and sodium. Maintains correct water balances in the system and prevents oedema, in conjunction with sodium. Helps maintain heart rhythm, correct blood pressure, and glandular functions.	Unsulphured dried fruits, soya flour, soya beans, molasses, raw nuts, wholegrains, all green leafy vegetables especially parsley, spinach, green beans, asparagus, lettuce, celery, onions, carrots, beetroot (raw as far as possible), raw egg yolk*, cheese, bananas, peaches, grapes and fish.
Selenium	Is an antioxidant like vitamins C and E, upon which it has a sparing effect and along with them is considered to be a protective factor against cancer.	Dried brewers' yeast, liver, brain, heart, kidney, seafoods, muscle meat, kelp, wholegrains, brazil nuts, garlic, milk, eggs and mushrooms.
Silicon Found in nature as silica (Silicon acid).	Strengthens teeth and bones in conjunction with calcium and phosphorous. Helps prevent brittle bones and soft teeth in conjunction with fluorine. Helps glandular systems clear waste matter from the body. Stimulates hair growth and a healthy and complexion.	Wholegrains, nuts, raw egg yolk*, sunflower seeds, apples, strawberries, grapes, cherries, peaches, raw cabbage, carrots, green leafy vegetables, including spinach, celery, beetroot, parsnips, turnips, leeks, cucumbers and tomatoes. Found in or just under skins or outer part of vegetables and fruits.
Sodium	Essential ingredient in tissue structure and for absorption of iron, calcium, potassium and fluorine. Sodium and potassium act together to keep the correct balance of body fluids (potassium in the cells and sodium in the fluids). Must be taken in its whole form as found in nature (in foods and sea salt) but not as refined table salt (sodium chloride) which is in a form the body cannot utilise correctly.	Egg yolk, condensed milk, cheese, white fish, raw nuts, wholegrains, apples, strawberries, peaches, figs, gooseberries, unsulphured dried fruits, lettuce, celery, carrots, turnips, cucumber, asparagus, spinach and beetroot. *Note:* Not the same as sodium chloride (table salt), an excess of which would result in excess liquid in tissues.
Sulphur	Essential ingredient of hair, nails, insulin and bile salts. Purifies system of toxins and improves tone of nervous system.	Raw egg yolk*, cheese, lean beef, wheat germ, lentils, peanuts, also cabbage, onions, turnips and radishes especially if eaten raw.

*Since the outbreak of salmonella poisoning in 1988 the Government has recommended that raw egg and recipes containing it should be avoided.

Nutrient	Functions	Good sources
Zinc	Essential for production of insulin, interrelated with vitamin B1 metabolism. Assists in digestion of protein and carbohydrates. Helps to speed healing of wounds and burns including infections such as colds. Essential for a healthy nervous system (exerts a balancing effect) hair, nails, skin, bones, kidney, pituitary gland and male reproductive organs. Thought to prevent absorption of cadmium (a toxic element).	Dried brewers' yeast, meat (especially liver), nuts, seeds, (especially pumpkin and sunflower), wheat germ, eggs, fish, (especially herring and oysters). *Note:* Zinc is lost through sweating and phytic acid in the diet and exposure to cadmium in cigarette smoke and car exhaust fumes.

Little known minerals

Elements	Details
Molybdenum	Can be found particularly in buckwheat, lima beans, wheat germ, liver, soya beans, barley, lentils, oats, sunflower seeds. A lack is thought to be linked with irregular heart beat, with irritability and tooth decay. Excessive amounts of molybdenum may be a factor contributing to gout and high blood levels of uric acid in areas of molybdenum rich soil.
Nickel	Found in buckwheat, oats, legumes and green leafy vegetables. A lack may be one of the factors associated with cirrhosis of the liver. In very small amounts nickel is thought to help stabilise the production of Deoxyribonucleic acid (DNA) and Ribonucleic acid (RNA). In tobacco, nickel combines with carbon monoxide to form the toxic nickel carbonyl which may be a factor in causing lung cancer. Acute effects of toxic nickel carbonyl include frontal headache, vertigo, vomiting, chest pain and cough. Note: DNA – a molecule in each cell that contains the blueprint for replication of that cell. RNA – another molecule (working in conjunction with DNA) assembles materials needed for repair and replacement of each cell.
Strontium	Found in the same foods as calcium and is stored in the bones. It may help to prevent tooth decay and osteoporosis. The only toxic form of strontium is strontium-90 the radioactive form produced by the effect of nuclear explosions.
Vanadium	Found in such foods as parsley, lobster, radish, dill and lettuce. Function little known but thought to help control cholesterol levels. Excessive amounts of vanadium may be related to manic depression.

Undesirable mineral elements

Lead, Cadmium and Mercury	Particularly toxic. Fish caught in inshore-polluted water may be contaminated by lead and methyl mercury. Other sources of mercury (apart from industrial exposure) include dental amalgam (eroded from tooth fillings), pesticides, paints and cosmetics. Mercury can produce symptoms of fatigue, forgetfulness and headaches. Vegetables and grains should be washed carefully as they are likely to be polluted by particles of lead and cadmium from industrial fallout or traffic fumes. Some fruits may have been sprayed with pesticides containing lead or mercury. Cigarette smoke contains traces of lead and cadmium; glazes and pigments used on some pottery may also contain lead and cadmium, which can leach out if the pottery is used to store foods such as acid fruit juices. Other sources of lead include petrol, lead pipes and lead-based paint. Lead toxicity is associated with hyperactivity and aggressive behaviour, especially in children, poor memory and poor concentration; Cadmium toxicity is associated with emphysema, anaemia, scaly skin, and loss of hair and kidney damage. Cadmium interferes with the body's absorption of calcium, copper, iron and zinc.
Aluminium	Considered non-toxic by saucepan manufactures but it is corroded by either acid or alkaline foods and is dissolved in water. There are also reports of persistent gastric troubles and skin troubles, which disappeared after stopping the use of aluminium utensils and returned when they were used again. Aluminium's function in the body is not known but it is used in foil, as an emulsifier. In some processed cheeses, cigarette filters, some tooth pastes and cosmetics, table salt and acids and other pharmaceutical products. Signs of aluminium toxicity include poor calcium metabolism (leading to the possibility of rickets in children and osteomalacia in adults), dermatitis, mental retardation and it may be a factor in senile dementia and Alzheimer's disease.
Arsenic	In very small amounts appears to be necessary for the health of animals but its specific functions are not known. Arsenic is found in some shellfish and meat (used in some animal foods) also in insecticides, cigarettes, glue and some beers. Although arsenic is readily excreted from the body, possible symptoms include intense thirst, aching muscles, tingling or numbness in the hands and feet, if there is no more obvious cause.
Sodium fluoride	Added to drinking water, some toothpastes and mouth rinses, for preventing tooth decay. It is an industrial by-product and thought to be toxic in large doses. It is quite different chemically from calcium fluoride found naturally in nature. Chronic long-term effects include acne, under active thyroid and hypersensitivity.

Supplementation with vitamins A, B6, C, E, the minerals calcium, magnesium, manganese, selenium and zinc, and the sulphur-containing amino acids cysteine and methionine, will help to detoxify the body. Calcium helps remove aluminium, cadmium and lead. Vitamin C effectively removes arsenic, aluminium and cadmium and helps to remove any excess nickel. Selenium can protect the body from arsenic and mercury; zinc is good at reducing levels of cadmium and lead and, to some extent, aluminium. The sulphur-containing amino acids cysteine and methionine found in such foods as garlic, onions and eggs protect against cadmium, lead and mercury toxicity. Vitamin B6, magnesium and, to some extent, manganese also help to remove aluminium from the system. Vitamin E helps to lower nickel levels, also arsenic and cadmium as do vitamin A along with vitamin C and selenium. In addition to calcium and zinc, exposure to cadmium may create a need for iron and copper supplementation since cadmium interferes with the absorption of all these nutrients.

Index